General Pathology
for Veterinary Nurses

Harriet Brooks
BVetMed, MSc, PhD, MRCVS, FHEA
Royal Veterinary College, North Mymms, Herts

WILEY-BLACKWELL

A John Wiley & Sons Ltd., Publication

Blackwell Publishing was acquired by John Wiley & Sons in February 2007.
Blackwell's publishing programme has been merged with Wiley's global Scientific,
Technical, and Medical business to form Wiley-Blackwell.

Registered office
John Wiley & Sons Ltd, The Atrium, Southern Gate, Chichester, West Sussex,
PO19 8SQ, United Kingdom

Editorial offices
9600 Garsington Road, Oxford, OX4 2DQ, United Kingdom
2121 State Avenue, Ames, Iowa 50014-8300, USA

For details of our global editorial offices, for customer services and for
information about how to apply for permission to reuse the copyright material in
this book please see our website at www.wiley.com/wiley-blackwell.

Library of Congress Cataloging-in-Publication Data

Brooks, Harriet W.
  General pathology for veterinary nurses / Harriet W. Brooks.
    p. ; cm.
  Includes index.
  ISBN 978-1-4051-5590-8 (pbk. : alk. paper)
  1. Veterinary pathology.   2. Veterinary nursing.   I. Title.
    [DNLM: 1. Animal Diseases–physiopathology–Nurses' Instruction.
  2. Pathology, Veterinary–Nurses' Instruction.   SF 774.5 B873g 2010]
    SF774.5.B76 2010
    636.089′607–dc22

                                                    2009027991

A catalogue record for this book is available from the British Library.

Set in 10/12.5pt Avenir by Aptara® Inc., New Delhi, India

1 2010

Contents

About This Book   v
Dedication   ix
Acknowledgements   x

1   Introduction to Veterinary Pathology   1

What is pathology?   2
Who 'does' pathology?   3
Pathology as an academic subject   9

2   Aetiology   11

Introduction   12
Aetiology – the study of the causes of disease   13

3   Cell Injury   23

Lesions – structural and functional changes   24
Definitions of cell response or injury following
    harmful stimulus   24
Cellular degeneration   26
Cell death – necrosis   30
Extracellular changes   35

4   Inflammation   41

What is inflammation?   42
Acute inflammation   43
Chronic inflammation   55

5 Pathology and the Immune System   65

The normal immune system   66
Diseases of the immune system   84

6 Tissue Repair   97

Definition of tissue repair or healing   98
Tissue repair – general and specific examples   103
Healing in various tissues   108
Healing regulation and control   109
What can impair, prevent or alter healing?   109

7 Circulatory Disorders   113

The normal circulatory system   114
Oedema   122
Impaired blood supply to tissues   127
Clotting (coagulation) of blood   132
Shock   145

8 Disorders of Cell/Tissue Growth   153

Atrophy, hypertrophy, hyperplasia and metaplasia   154
Neoplasia   157

Glossary   189
Answers to Test Yourself Questions   215
Further Reading   237
Index   239

About This Book

Don't skip this part! This section will explain how to get the most from this book.

Aims of this section

- To introduce general pathology
- To explain the format of the book
- To give some general information

Welcome to general pathology!

What do we mean by general pathology? Before answering that, let us talk about pathology in its broadest sense.

What is pathology to you?

You may think of pathologists as people in paper suits, who get involved with murder investigations on the television, very remote from your everyday life. If you are already studying for your nursing qualification, you may view pathology as a dreary subject to be passed on the way to the more exciting subjects of surgical or medical nursing. You may have completed your studies and feel you 'got by' without needing to know too much pathology anyway.

Well, I hope that, through this book, I can help you to view pathology as not so boring after all, and relevant to every one of us involved in veterinary medicine.

Pathology underpins all you do as a veterinary nurse; it is central to veterinary science. Apart from some elective surgical procedures, all that exciting medicine and surgery hinge on pathological processes occurring within the body. Understanding these pathological processes will help you to understand the clinical presentations of your patients, to follow the rationale of the treatments used in the clinics, and to explain the conditions and procedures to anxious owners. A good understanding of pathology will turn a competent veterinary nurse into an outstanding one.

So, what is pathology?

This question will be answered more fully in the first two chapters, but briefly, pathology is the study of the effects of disease on the body. It is a broad subject, encompassing a number of sub-divisions such as *general* pathology, *systematic* (or *special*) pathology and *clinical* pathology.

This book concentrates on general pathology, which is the study of the basic pathological processes that are not specific to particular organs or tissues. For instance, processes such as cell degeneration, inflammation and tumour formation are pretty much the same in all parts of the body, and so are considered under the heading of general pathology.

Other textbooks and references will cover *systematic* pathology, discussing specific organ systems. If you refer to these texts you will be able to apply the knowledge of general pathology that you gain from this book.

Clinical (or *chemical*) *pathology* is the pathology used in the laboratory, whether the practice laboratory or a diagnostic laboratory – many general nursing texts cover basic clinical pathology, e.g. urinalysis or blood biochemistry, so I have not covered these aspects in this book.

The format of this book and how to use it

Each chapter starts with two boxes, one giving an outline of the chapter and the other explaining the aims of the chapter. Read the aims box carefully. Understanding the aims of each chapter will help to guide your reading of the topic.

There are sub-headings dividing up each chapter into main topics and at the end of each chapter is another text box summarising the main points covered in the chapter.

More boxes!

Dotted through the text there are diagrams and tables and a few photographs, all included as numbered boxes. These numbered boxes aim to summarise information or revise it, so that many important topics will be encountered three times – in the text, in the diagram and as a caption to the diagram. The diagrams and tables can also be used as a revision aid if you are unlucky enough to be facing examinations. A glossary of terms used in the book, or that you may come across in your reading, is included towards the back of the book.

You might find that some areas do not have summary boxes when you feel you could do with them or a useful term is omitted from the glossary; in this case, draw up your own boxes to help your study and add missing words to the glossary – do not just accept what I have given you! Remember this book is just a starting point for you – use it to gain the basics and the confidence to start to read around the subject. Who knows where you could end up?

Questions, questions!

Each chapter finishes with up to six test yourself questions. The questions vary slightly in their format and some require short snappy answers, whilst others could almost require short essay answers. These are to help you make sure you have understood what you have read; use them in whatever way helps you most. You may like to actually sit and write your answers from memory, you may like to jot notes or key words or you may find just reading through the questions helps you. At the end of the book are some suggested answers; however, you choose to use the questions, try not to cheat! It will help you most if you have a go at answering the questions yourself before you read my suggestions.

The book is designed to be a workbook. If this is your own book, do not be afraid to personalise it – jot notes or reminders in the margin, cross reference to published articles or to other parts of the book, or to cases you have seen in the clinics. Annotate the diagrams; draw moustaches on the cartoons. Make this book totally yours. (Note – do not do this if it is a library copy, if you are reading this in a bookshop or if it belongs to someone else.)

Your roles

You will need to be an active reader to get the most from this book! Many sections within this book build on one another. Some prior knowledge of histology, anatomy and physiology is expected, so you may need to refer to other texts or study notes to supplement some areas if you are uncertain what is being discussed.

Get in touch – the author would like to hear from you if you have comments or complaints, or suggestions for future editions.

Most of all, I hope you will enjoy reading and using this book and that it might change your mind about pathology (unless, of course you liked it all along!).

This book is dedicated to my parents, with fondest love

Acknowledgements

I am indebted first and foremost to Wiley-Blackwell for inviting me to write this book, and thanks to many people there, but especially Katy Loftus, for encouragement, advice and extreme patience during its protracted production.

Many thanks also to all of my family, especially my mother and husband, for their support, love and a good deal of humour; I might have given up many times had you not all kept me going. Thanks also to Joe, my husband, for comments on Chapter 5, and for the use of his photograph in that chapter, and to Helen Wakeham for allowing us to photograph her sow and piglets.

My beloved canine companions – Daisy, Dilly and Edie – deserve a mention for keeping my spirits high and for taking me out for many a good walk to clear my mind.

This book is based on my pathology teaching material for trainee nurses at the Royal Veterinary College. So finally, but certainly not least, I acknowledge all past and future trainee veterinary nurses who have inspired me to write the book; I truly hope it helps to underpin your chosen careers, and I wish you every happiness and success in the future.

Harriet Brooks

Chapter 1

Introduction to Veterinary Pathology

What is pathology?

Who 'does' pathology?

    Anatomic pathology
    Clinical pathology
    Microbiology
    Parasitology
    Immunology
    Toxicology
    Veterinary forensic pathology
    Government agency laboratories
    Pharmaceutical laboratories

Pathology as an academic subject

Aims of Chapter 1

- To define pathology as part of (veterinary) medicine
- To define general pathology as part of pathology
- To briefly discuss how pathology is used everyday, and who uses it and where it is used

---

What is pathology?

The word pathology comes from two Greek words, *Pathos* – which literally means *'experience'* or *'something which one suffers'*, but which in this context is used in terms of suffering *from a disease*, and *-logy* meaning *'word'*, *'speech'* or *'reason'*. The suffix *-logy* is used in compound words (when it is added to another word such as in biology, physiology and entomology), and then it infers *'study of'* or *'science of'*.

So, *pathology is the branch of medical science that involves study of the causes of diseases, how they develop and their effects on the body.* It encompasses any deviation from a healthy or normal condition in any living creature. There is even a branch of horticulture that involves study of pathology in plants.

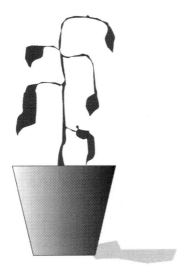

In pathology, the effects of diseases can be studied at various levels: the *whole body*, the *organs* or *tissues*, *cells* and even *within cells* (at sub-cellular level) (see Box 1.1).

Box 1.1 What is pathology?

Pathology is the branch of medical science involving study of the *causes* of diseases, how they *develop* and their *effects* on the body.

Pathology includes consideration of any deviation from a healthy or normal condition, in any living creature (including plants).

In pathology, the effects of diseases are studied at various levels: the *whole body*, the *organs* or *tissues*, the *cells* and even *within cells* (at sub-cellular level).

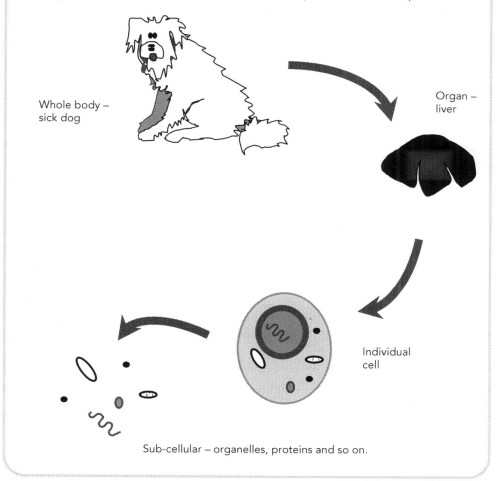

Whole body – sick dog

Organ – liver

Individual cell

Sub-cellular – organelles, proteins and so on.

Who 'does' pathology?

You might answer that question by saying pathologists do, and that is certainly correct. We will discuss pathologists in a moment, but the 'pathologically trained' professionals are not the only ones actively engaged in pathology. If you are working in general practice, you are too.

As we said at the beginning of this chapter, pathology involves not just study of what causes diseases, but also how diseases develop and their effects on the body. Every time you record the temperature, pulse and respiration of a patient, use a dipstick to test an animal's urine, run an automated blood analyser, change the dressing on an infected wound, or advise an owner about flea control to help their cat's red itchy skin, or diet to control diarrhoea in a sensitive golden retriever, you are assessing the deviation from a healthy or normal condition in the animal; you are assessing pathological changes. So, you and the vets, physiotherapists and others with whom you work use their knowledge of pathology. But there will be times when you require help from a pathology diagnostic laboratory to make the diagnosis; perhaps you need tests beyond the scope of your practice laboratory.

Pathology laboratories may be independent businesses, or they may be based at a university veterinary school, or they may be government agencies. The pathologists who work at these laboratories are often classified according to the type of diagnostic work they do, though a few will be all-rounders and will do everything!

Anatomic pathology

Anatomic pathologists study disease by looking at tissue and organs. This may be by performing post-mortem examinations (also called *necropsies*) and writing a post-mortem report, or by looking at tissues from live animals (called *biopsies*). Anatomic pathologists will look at the tissues or organs by eye (gross examination) to identify abnormalities, but also use histologic sections, mounted on glass slides to look at the tissue under the microscope (see Box 1.2).

Clinical pathology

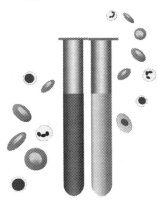

Clinical pathologists assess disease in an animal by studying body fluids (such as blood, urine, joint fluid, abdominal tap fluid, cerebrospinal fluid and so on). They may look at the chemical composition (*clinical biochemistry*) or the types of cells in the fluid or in an FNA, using a microscope to study a stained smear of the sample on a glass microscope slide (this is called *cytology*). Clinical pathologists might spot bacteria or other infectious organisms in a cytology preparation.

Box 1.2 How histology sections are produced (see diagram below)

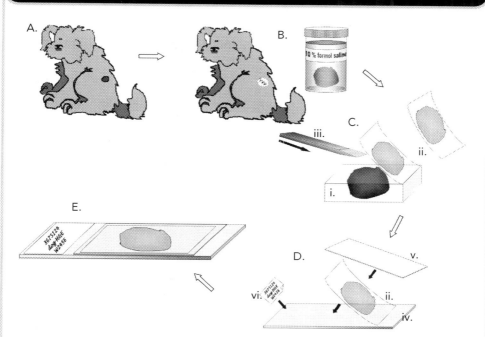

A. A dog is presented at the vet's surgery with a skin tumour.

B. Taking a biopsy, the vet decides to remove the tumour, perhaps after performing a fine-needle aspirate (FNA) and checking what the mass is. The vet and owner decide that they would like to send the mass to a pathologist to confirm the diagnosis. The mass is placed in a fixative solution which will preserve the tissue by fixing (denaturing) the proteins. Usually, a 10% solution of formalin is used (10% formol saline). In this example, the vet has removed (excised) the whole mass, this is called an *excision biopsy*. Sometimes only a part of a tissue is removed (incisional biopsy) and sent for histopathology. The biopsy is sent to the laboratory in a leakproof, wide-mouthed container.

C. In the laboratory, the tissue is *processed* by embedding it in a paraffin wax block (i). When this is done, very thin, almost transparent, slices of the tissue can be taken (ii), using an extremely sharp cutting instrument, called a *microtome* (iii). These slices are so thin that 1 cm of tissue could be sliced 5000 times.

D. A thin slice of the tissue is placed flat (*mounted*) on a glass microscope slide (iv), and dyed using histological stains. The standard staining method uses the stains haematoxylin and eosin (often shortened to 'H and E') which stains the sections pink and blue. The stains allow the pathologist to examine the tissues more easily than would an unstained section. The tissue section is protected by

> **Box 1.2** (*Continued*) How histology sections are produced
>
> a very thin glass *cover slip* (v) which is glued on top. Finally, the slide is labelled with a reference number and other laboratory details (vi).
>
> E. The pathologist examines the tissue section under the microscope and writes a report, which may suggest a diagnosis and prognosis. In the case of our dog's tumour, the pathologist may also be able to tell whether the vet has managed to remove it all or whether further surgery at the site is advisable (the pathologist can tell this by looking at the edges of the tumour and observing whether there is a rim of normal tissue around the edge – the *excision margins*).

Haematology is specifically the study of cell types in blood, and this can indicate an increase in white blood cells (*leucocytes*) in an animal fighting an infection or a decrease in red blood cells (*erythrocytes*) in an animal with anaemia.

An anatomic or clinical pathologist may suspect that infectious organisms are involved in the disease and may suggest a fresh (unfixed) sample should be sent for *microbiology* (see below) if the practice has not already done this.

Microbiology

Microbiologists study *infectious organisms* that may be associated with diseases, more specifically, bacteriologists study bacteria, virologists study viruses, and mycologists study fungi and yeasts. Clinical samples, such as urine, pus, mucus or even tissue may be sent to microbiology laboratories where they have the equipment, skills and expertise to grow (*culture*) and identify infectious organisms. In the case of bacterial infection, they may also be able to assess which antibiotics the organism is likely to be killed by (the *sensitivity* of the organism) which gives the vet an indication of what treatment to use.

Parasitology

Although the very small creatures studied by microbiologists could be described as being parasitic, parasitologists tend to be associated with the study of slightly larger organisms which live on or in other animals. So, parasitology encompasses the study of, for instance, parasitic worms in the gut, fleas living on the skin or demodex mites living in hair follicles.

Immunology

Sometimes an infectious organism is suspected of causing disease in an animal, but that organism itself cannot be cultured in the microbiology laboratory or seen in samples under the microscope. In this case, the immunology laboratory may be able to tell whether the animal has been infected by the suspected organism by looking for *antibodies*. Antibodies are produced by the body's immune system to help fight disease (this is part of what is known as an *immune response*); specific antibodies are produced for specific infectious agents, so finding certain antibodies will indicate that an animal has come into contact with a certain infectious agent (or has responded to a vaccine).

Infectious organisms have proteins on their surfaces, called *antigens*. These antigens are a sort of 'fingerprint' which the immune system can usually recognise as being 'foreign' and this stimulates the immune response. Sometimes specific antigens can be detected in samples by immunological tests.

Such immunological tests may be done on blood *serum* (this is called *serology*). Some immunological tests can also be carried out on tissues mounted on microscope slides, and this is then known as *immunostaining*. All types of cells of the body have their own 'fingerprint', though in a healthy individual the immune system recognises these and doesn't start to react against them. Sometimes we can use this property of cells to confirm the diagnosis, for instance, if a pathologist is having trouble identifying a particular skin tumour under the microscope immunostains for specific cell types can be applied to the tissue and can help to reveal the identity of the tumour.

Toxicology

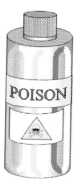

In some cases, toxicologists may be asked to analyse samples for toxins or poisons, for instance, you or the pathologist might send stomach contents, urine or even fresh tissue from a necropsy in the case of an animal suspected of being poisoned. The laboratory may need some guidance as to which toxic substance is suspected, such as a reliable history of known or likely contact of an animal with that particular substance. Note also that very often the toxins or poisons break down or are metabolised after having their damaging effects, and may not be detected in biological samples. In these cases, the animal presents with clinical signs that require diagnosis and treatment, such as a severely anaemic animal that has eaten anticoagulant rodent poison. The priority is to treat the anaemia, and toxicology may not be helpful, though it could be argued that confirming the cause of the animal's signs may help to prevent poisoning in other animals.

Veterinary forensic pathology

There are a small number of veterinary pathologists who deal with forensic cases; that is, cases where there may be suggestions of cruelty or malicious harm to men or animals, or police involvement due to suspected illegal activity of one sort or another. This subject is beyond the scope of this book, and it is usually best for general practices to seek advice if they get drawn into such a case unless they are experienced in dealing with them. As a rule of thumb all those involved with the case, including veterinary nurses, may be asked to give evidence at a later stage, and should always keep notes, photographs, logged telephone calls or case records securely and safely stored, in case they need to submit them to the authorities as part of the investigation. Any biological material, including bodies of deceased animals, should be logged and labelled, and stored securely until removal by an authorised person.

Government agency laboratories

Some pathologists are employed as veterinary investigation officers, and work for government agency laboratories. These laboratories principally investigate diseases in farm or production animals. As well as investigating disease in individual or small groups of animals, these pathologists are important in helping to maintain herd or flock health on farms and nationally. This helps to prevent widespread infectious diseases and to protect our food quality (and safety) and human health.

Pharmaceutical laboratories

Veterinary pathologists work at pharmaceutical laboratories too. Here they will help to investigate diseases and to develop drugs to treat men and animals. They will also take an interest in apparent unexpected drug reactions.

Pathology as an academic subject

This chapter has so far discussed some of the ways pathology is carried out in practice and who undertakes it. Pathology is a broad academic subject, and when we study it, we often divide it into *general* pathology and *systematic* (or *special*) pathology. What does this mean?

- *General* pathology is the study of *processes in disease*, without necessarily limiting discussion to one particular tissue or organ. For instance, inflammation and neoplasia are general pathological processes.
- Whereas *systematic* (special) pathology is the study of the *effects of disease* with *special reference to a specific tissue* or *a body system*. For instance, dermatitis (inflammation in the skin) and osteosarcoma (neoplasia of bone) are examples of systematic or special pathological changes.

From now on this book focuses on general pathology, but we will use examples of specific organs or body systems to help you understand the processes we are discussing, and perhaps to relate the topic to diseases you may have encountered in general veterinary practice.

Summary of key points in Chapter 1

- Pathology is the study of the causes of diseases, of how they develop and their effects on the body. It encompasses any deviation from a healthy or normal condition in any living creature.
- Veterinary pathology is carried out by a number of different people, from nurses and vets in general practice to trained pathologists in academia or industry.
- General pathology is the study of *processes* in disease, without limiting discussion to a particular tissue or organ. Inflammation and neoplasia are examples of general pathological processes.
- Systematic (special) pathology is the study of general pathology processes but with special reference to specific tissues or body systems, for instance, dermatitis (inflammation in the skin) and osteosarcoma (neoplasia of bone) are examples of systematic or special pathological changes.

Test yourself questions on Chapter 1

1. What is meant by the term 'pathology'?
2. Briefly discuss the work of
   a. anatomic pathologists and
   b. clinical pathologists.
3. a. What organisms are studied by microbiologists? (*list as many types as you can*)
   b. Still thinking about microbiology, what is meant by 'sensitivity' and why is it helpful and/or important?
4. Briefly suggest some sensible actions to take if you are involved in a case which involves the police or other authorities.
5. Why are veterinary pathologists important for the health of human beings?
6. What is meant by 'general' pathology and how does it differ from 'systematic' or 'special' pathology?

Chapter 2
Aetiology

Introduction to aetiology

Aetiology – the study of the causes of disease

What are aetiological agents?
Classification of aetiological agents
Classification of diseases
What determines whether disease occurs?

Aims of Chapter 2

- To define the term aetiology and discuss the main types of aetio-logical agents
- To discuss other factors which may act with aetiological agents in the development of disease
- To consider the main ways in which aetiological agents cause disease

Introduction to aetiology

Let us start with a few terms you may come across in your reading. Aetiology is pronounced *eet-ee-ology*. In American textbooks you may see it spelt without the first 'a' – *etiology*, but it is still pronounced as above.

You would have spotted that aetiology is another compound word (like the word pathology, discussed in Chapter 1) in which '-*logy*' denotes '*study of*' or '*science of*'. The first part comes from the Greek word '*aitia*' meaning 'cause'. So, aetiology means *the study or science of the causes of disease*.

The word *pathogenesis* is associated with aetiology. Pathogenesis involves '*pathos*' again, as introduced in Chapter 1, but in this case it is linked with *genesis*, which comes from the Greek verb for '*to become*' or '*to produce, to bring forth*'. Thus, pathogenesis relates to *things which produce disease*, and tends to be used when discussing how factors *lead to disease*, or *the mechanisms of disease development*. It describes the chain of events from the initial stimulus to the manifestation of the disease or the lesion produced.

There are some other terms we use which relate to pathogenesis. A factor which is capable of producing disease may be referred to as *pathogenic*, and an infectious agent (bacteria, virus and fungus) capable of causing disease may often be referred to in non-specific terms as a *pathogen*. The term *aetiological agent* is also used for a factor capable of causing disease.

Do not worry too much about these terms at this stage; you will become more familiar with their usage as you read through this book and other texts.

So, now we have got some definitions out of the way; let us start to discuss aetiology.

Aetiology – the study of the causes of disease

Diseases occur when a harmful trigger (of whatever type) causes loss of normal health or disrupts a tissue or organ. Many diseases tend to have distinct and recognisable cause(s) (aetiology), development processes (pathogenesis), lesions and clinical signs.

Let us consider a familiar example to illustrate this. Two cats have a fight, and a few days later one of them develops an abscess in the skin on its back. Now think about the features of diseases in turn and apply them to our cat:

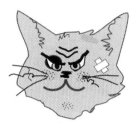

Cause(s): bacteria from one cat's mouth are introduced into another cat's skin via the teeth.

Development process: the bacteria multiply and start up the process of inflammation in the skin of the bitten cat. Inflammatory cells and bacteria die and accumulate as a pool of pus[1], with a rim of active inflammation around it (an abscess).

Lesion: surface skin wound and scab; abscess in the skin; heat (due to inflammation).

Clinical signs: pain, heat, swelling, pus, depression, loss of appetite, grumpiness etc.

In other cases it may be harder to clearly define diseases in this way. Many diseases involve more than one cause (aetiological agent), or they may be made more complex by other factors such as secondary infections. Development processes may be altered by other concurrent diseases. Finally, especially in veterinary patients, the lesions and clinical signs are often complicated by self-trauma – the animal licking, biting or scratching a diseased area, for instance.

We now go on to discuss some of the aetiological agents and some of the complicating factors that can affect disease development.

---

[1] Pus = thick fluid sometimes formed as a result of inflammation, consisting of white blood cells (especially neutrophils, see Chapter 4), dead cells and often also containing living and dead bacteria. By the way, note the correct spelling. Examiners HATE to see it referred to as 'puss'!

What are aetiological agents?

We said above that aetiological agents are factors capable of causing disease or tissue damage. Our knowledge of aetiological agents has altered as our scientific understanding has increased. In historical times, evil spirits, bad humors and foul smells were all considered to cause disease. Old rags were thought to cause bubonic plague (the Black Death) during medieval times – it was actually fleas on rats living in the rags which carried the plague bacterium.

The first microscopes were developed in the second half of the 1600s, allowing closer study of tissues and even description of bacteria, though the role of bacteria in disease was not recognised for another 200 years or so. Rudimentary, though successful, attempts at vaccination for diseases we now know to be caused by viruses, such as smallpox, were carried out from the 1770s.

Yeasts and fungi were first recognised for their roles in fermentation, and later some types of these organisms were found to be involved in disease especially in patients with weakened immune systems. The roles of nutrition and hygiene started to be taken seriously in the late 1800s and continued to gather momentum since then. By 1855, it was realised that a cholera outbreak in London was linked to a particular supply of drinking water in Lambeth, and since then our understanding of the infectious and environmental factors involved in disease development and tissue injury has grown enormously.

Sadly, the great wars have added to our understanding of physical trauma (but also have clearly illustrated the importance of emergency nursing for longer-term prognosis). More recently, molecular biology has increased our knowledge of the DNA in our genes; this has helped us to recognise the genetic basis of some diseases.

Throughout this book, we shall tend to consider aetiological agents in general terms, though we shall use a few specific examples to illustrate pathological processes. Other textbooks will be the sources of more specific information on causes of particular diseases (see Further Reading, page 238).

Classification of aetiological agents

To help our understanding we can usefully classify aetiological agents in various ways. You may see other classifications in other textbooks,

Box 2.1 Classification of aetiological agents

Internal factors

- Genetic – *defects* or *mutations*
- Immune system – *defects* or *abnormal responses*
- Aging – *natural* processes or premature aging

External factors

- Physical – *trauma, pressure* etc.
- Chemical – *toxins, poisons, heavy metals* etc.
- Infectious – *parasites, bacteria, viruses, fungi* etc.
- Environmental – *nutrition* (*deficiencies or excesses*)
    - *temperature*
    - *hygiene*
    - *radiation, e.g. ultraviolet light*

but a helpful start is to consider aetiological agents as internal or external factors, such as in Box 2.1.

Think about the table in Box 2.1 – does it work for you?

You might wish to slightly reclassify some items, for instance, in external factors (the bottom half of the table), physical and chemical factors could be classified under environmental factors. Or temperature of the environment could be considered a physical factor. Should hormones be included in the list of internal factors, after all they have detrimental effects in disorders like hyperadrenocorticism (Cushing's disease) and diabetes mellitus?

Do not be afraid to annotate or draw up your own version of this table as you read on through this book!

Classification of diseases

Diseases can broadly be considered as follows.

Acquired diseases

These are diseases which develop at some stage during life, as a result of the effects of one or more aetiological agent acting during life.

Examples of acquired diseases would be pneumonia or dermatitis due to fleas.

Congenital diseases

These are diseases which the animal or person is born with. Congenital diseases occur because the aetiological agent acts on the developing embryo or foetus, on the uterus or placenta, or on the mother, either before or during pregnancy. Note that clinical signs of a congenital disease may not be seen at birth, but may show up later in life. They are still called congenital and not acquired because the aetiological agent actually had its effect before birth.

Developmental abnormalities, such as heart defects, and forms of muscular dystrophy in certain dog breeds, such as golden retrievers, would be examples of congenital diseases (see Box 2.2).

Some diseases, notably cancers, are a bit more difficult to divide up this way as they may involve both congenital and hereditary damage to genes *and* exposure to some factor(s) during life to start the cancer growing (see section on Neoplasia in Chapter 8). In diseases involving both acquired and congenital phases, we consider that the initial congenital gene mutation has made that individual *susceptible* to later diseases if he or she comes into contact with a suitable *trigger factor* during life.

Idiopathic diseases

There are some diseases of which we do not (yet) know the cause, though they may have recognisable development processes, lesions or clinical signs. These are diseases we refer to as *idiopathic.*

What determines whether disease occurs?

Simple diseases

If a disease has an uncomplicated development that could be summarised as:

$$\text{aetiological agent} + \text{tissue} = \text{disease}$$

it would be known as a *simple* disease (see Box 2.3).

In reality, there are few diseases or disorders which are this uncomplicated, and in the vast majority of cases we need to consider what other factors act to make disease *more likely* to occur in the animal, or which *modify* the disease (for instance, factors which make the disease more severe or last longer in one animal compared with another). Factors associated with increasing likelihood of disease or which modify the course of a disease are shown in Box 2.4.

Multifactorial diseases

So, rather than being simple, as defined above, many diseases are more complicated and their course is affected or modified by lots of other factors and infectious agents. A good example of just such a

Box 2.2 Congenital versus hereditary diseases

People often get confused between *congenital* and *hereditary* diseases.

Congenital means a disease that is present at birth or develops due to the effects of some aetiological factor on the developing embryo or foetus, on the mother before or during pregnancy, or on the uterus or placenta.

Let us consider some hypothetical rabbits! Male and female hypothetical rabbit mate and the female gets pregnant. At some stage, either before or during her pregnancy she is exposed to or encounters a harmful stimulus (aetiological factor) of some type – it might be an infection or a poison, for instance. As a result of this some or, more likely, all of her babies from that litter are born with a hypothetical disease – let us say it makes their ears go spotty and drop off. Future litters of babies are not necessarily affected.

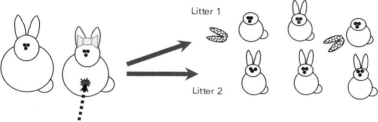

Aetiological factor acts on the developing baby, on the mother before or during pregnancy, or on the uterus or placenta of Litter 1.

As a result babies in Litter 1 are born with or develop *congenital* 'spotty-dropping-off'ear disease.

A *hereditary* condition is a disease or disorder that *can be passed on* from either or both parents to their offspring. More than one offspring may be affected, and successive offspring may also have the disease.

In this case, either the male or female hypothetical rabbits have a gene which leads to the hereditary disease in all those hypothetical baby rabbits who inherit the gene from either mum or dad. In this case, all future litters involving the parent who carries the gene may inherit the necessary gene and could be afflicted with the disorder. Some animals may carry the gene but not show the disease. (Note that this is a *very* simplified explanation to help to explain the difference between congenital and hereditary! Please consult more specific texts for further details of genetics if required.)

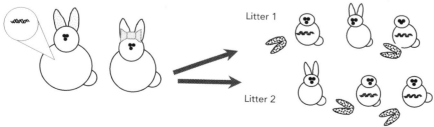

One of the parent hypothetical rabbits carries a gene which predisposes him to an inherited form of 'spotty-dropping-off' ear disease.

Baby rabbits who inherit the gene may also develop, or be born with, the inherited 'spotty-dropping-off' ear disease.

Box 2.3 Diagrammatic representation of a simple disease

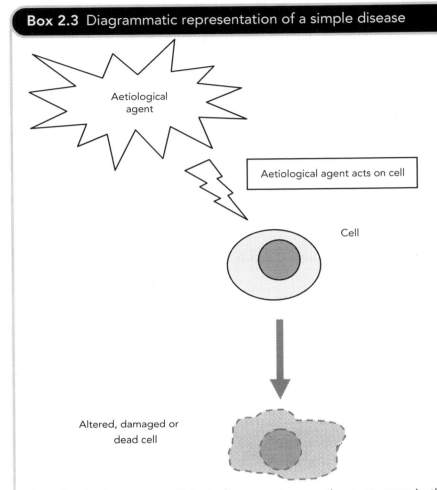

In a simple disease, an aetiological agent acts on a tissue or organ in the body (represented here by a very simplistic diagram of a cell). The aetiological agent causes cell damage or a change in normal function of the cell.

If many cells are affected the result is that the function of the whole organ, of which the cell is a part, is altered and consequently disease occurs in the animal.

A disease with such an uncomplicated development can be summarised as:

$$\text{aetiological agent} + \text{tissue} = \text{disease}$$

Box 2.4 Factors which make disease more likely to occur or which can modify the course of the disease

- **Age**   Often very young or old patients are more vulnerable to diseases
- **Immune system**   Lack of immunity in young, unvaccinated or naïve* animals, or any cause of reduced immunity in a previous immune animal will increase vulnerability to diseases
- **Genes**   A fault or mutation in a gene may make an animal more susceptible to the disease-causing agent
- **Other disease**   Having another disease already can often increase vulnerability by reducing the animal's ability to produce an immune response
- **Environmental factors**   Poor hygiene, extremes of temperature, mental stress, hunger, thirst, overcrowding etc. can increase vulnerability
- **Some drugs**   Certain drugs may affect the course of a disease, for instance, corticosteroids which may be used to reduce inflammation but can also limit immune responses and healing processes

*Naïve – pronounced 'ny-eeve'. This means animals who have not encountered a particular infectious agent before and so have not developed immunity to it.

multifactorial disease is canine infectious respiratory disease (CIRD) often called 'kennel cough' (see Box 2.5).

CIRD involves viruses and bacteria, but is also associated with various other factors, such as barking, housing in groups, age and so on; there is even a suggestion that certain breeds of dog are more vulnerable to contracting respiratory disease.

You can see that control, prevention and treatment of multifactorial diseases are somewhat more complicated than that for simple diseases, and veterinary professionals must consider many factors when giving advice or devising treatment and control plans.

So, this concludes a brief discussion of aetiology, or causal factors, of disease. In the next chapters, we look more at the responses, desired and harmful, of the body to these causal factors.

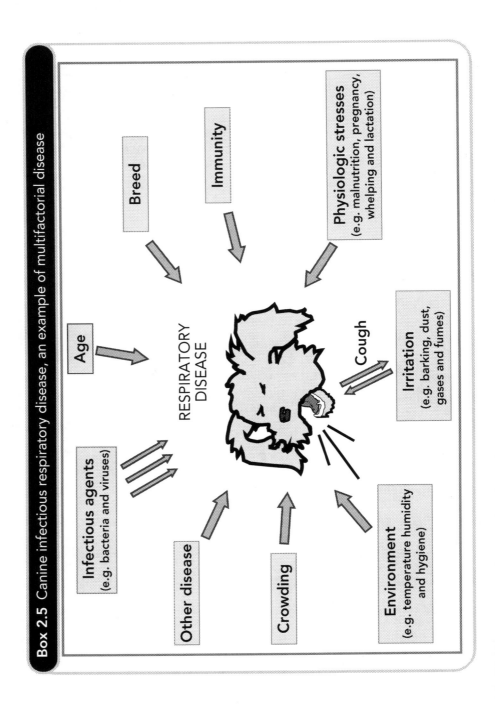

Box 2.5 Canine infectious respiratory disease, an example of multifactorial disease

Summary of key points in Chapter 2

- Aetiology is the study or science of the causes of disease, whereas the pathogenesis of a disease is how certain factors lead to the disease, or the mechanisms of disease development.
- A few diseases are simple in their pathogenesis – an aetiological agent causes disease.
- Many diseases are multifactorial – the animal is made more vulnerable to disease caused by the agent because of the effects of modifying factors (such as environment, age, nutrition, other infections etc.).

Test yourself questions on Chapter 2

1. What is meant by the term 'aetiology' (or etiology)?
2. What does it mean if a factor is described as 'pathogenic'?
3. Briefly discuss the classification of aetiological agents, including examples to illustrate your answer.
4. Write short notes to indicate the difference between (i) acquired diseases, (ii) congenital diseases and (iii) idiopathic diseases.
5. Suggest up to six factors which may modify the course of a multifactorial disease in an animal, including those factors which make disease more likely to occur in a particular animal.

Chapter 3
Cell Injury

Lesions – structural and functional changes

Definitions of cell response or injury following
harmful stimulus

Cellular degeneration

Cell death – necrosis

Types of necrosis
Sequelae of necrosis

Extracellular changes

Mineralisation
Crystals
Protein

> ### Aims of Chapter 3
>
> - To introduce the concept of structural and functional cell changes in response to harmful or injurious stimuli as the basis of gross pathological lesions
> - To define cell changes as reversible (for instance, adaptation and degeneration) or irreversible (such as cell death – necrosis), and to discuss commonly encountered examples of each
> - To discuss some common extracellular changes in tissues in response to various stimuli

Lesions – structural and functional changes

Lesions are *pathological changes* in tissues or organs. We think of lesions as abnormalities we can see, such as an area of abnormal colour on a liver or an ulcerated area on the skin; we call them *gross* lesions when we can see the abnormalities with the naked eye. But we need to remember that gross lesions are actually manifestations of abnormalities or changes *in the cells* which make up that tissue or organ (we can call these changes or abnormalities in cells *cellular lesions*). These changes in cells occur in response *to injurious*, that is harmful, *stimuli* (in other words, *aetiological agents*, see Chapter 2).

So, if abnormalities occur at the cellular level they are likely to lead to changes in tissue structure. The other effect they may have is to alter the *function* of the tissue, so for instance a harmful toxin that damages liver cells will, if enough liver cells are damaged, alter the function of the liver (as well as altering the look – colour, texture, size, shape – of the liver) (see Box 3.1).

You might think that there would be lots of different cellular responses to all the different harmful stimuli which may be encountered; in fact, there are only a few broad *categories* of cellular change (though there are lots of different effects on the animal depending which cells are affected). We shall discuss the cell changes in detail in this chapter and also in Chapter 8. You will find that these cell injuries will crop up throughout this book, so it is worth getting the hang of them at this stage.

We start by defining two important categories of cell changes in response to harmful stimuli – reversible and irreversible cell injury.

Definitions of cell response or injury following harmful stimulus

Reversible cell injury – cell injury causes alteration or loss of cell function and structural changes, but the cell *can* recover and regain structure

Box 3.1 Lesions – structural and functional changes

Lesions are *pathological changes* in tissues or organs. We think of lesions as abnormalities. When we can see the abnormalities with the naked eye we call them *gross lesions*.

Gross lesions are really manifestations of abnormalities or changes right down at the microscopic level – *in the cells* which make up that tissue or organ (i.e. *cellular lesions*).

Cellular lesions occur in response *to injurious* (harmful) *stimuli* (*aetiological agents*).

Abnormalities occurring at the cellular level can therefore cause changes in tissue structure, but also in the *function* of the tissue.

For instance, consider a busy liver cell. A harmful toxin comes into contact with this cell and causes harm to the cell in some way – perhaps it damages one of the tiny structures (organelles) within the cytoplasm which are important for the function of the cell. This damage is the cellular lesion.

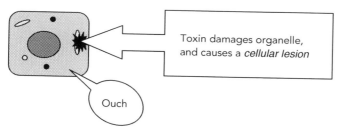

Toxin damages organelle, and causes a *cellular lesion*

Ouch

The cellular lesion affects the function of our liver cell and it will not be able to do its job properly, or may even die because of the lesion in its organelle. If lots of cells in the liver also come into contact with the toxin and all are similarly affected then the function of the liver as a whole may be affected, plus the look of the liver may be altered.

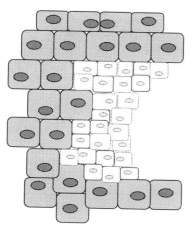

Toxin damages organelles of lots of cells, causing *cellular lesions* in them all.

As a result, the function of all these cells (shown in white) is impaired – thus, the function of the liver as a whole may be affected. In addition, the physical appearance of the liver may change. In this diagram, the affected cells have died as a result of their cellular lesions and have become pale and shrivelled. The gross lesion on the surface of the liver would be pale and sunken.

Cells do not always die and shrink; they can also become enlarged or change to another type of cell, for instance, but in so doing they can cause altered structure and function of the tissue as a whole.

and function if the injuring stimulus is removed. These are also called *sublethal* cell injuries/changes, that is 'not quite lethal' injuries.

Irreversible cell injury – cell injury causes alteration or loss of cell function and structural changes, but the cell *cannot* recover if the stimulus stops or is removed. In other words, the cell passes a 'point of no return' and even if the harmful stimulus stops, the cell will simply die (see *necrosis*) (see Box 3.2).

The *type* of change in the cell or tissue depends on a number of factors specific to the harmful stimulus and to the tissue itself; these are summarised in Box 3.3.

So to summarise, the cells' responses to injurious or harmful stimuli are:

- *Degeneration* – which is a reversible response.

But in the case of prolonged exposure of the cell to a harmful stimulus, or exposure to a very severe (large) stimulus, or if the cell has a poor blood supply, or in a cell with high metabolic rate, cellular degeneration may progress to:

- *Necrosis* – which is an irreversible response and the cell dies.

There are other changes which can occur which involve the cell responding (adapting) by

- *Changes in cell growth, size, number* – these can be either reversible *or* irreversible (see Chapter 8).

Box 3.8 includes a summary of all these cellular responses.

In this chapter, we will discuss the various types of cellular degeneration encountered in pathological lesions and then, what happens when cells die (necrosis).

Cellular degeneration

Cellular degenerations usually involve accumulation of substances within cells. There are various types of substances which may accumulate and the following discussion concerns some of the more common intracellular accumulations. In severe cases of the accumulations described below, the affected organ will become swollen and discoloured because so many (if not all) of the cells making up the organ are swollen with the accumulated substance (see Box 3.4).

- *Accumulation of cellular components*: As cells age, old and non-functional cellular components (organelles) may shrivel up or be

Box 3.2 Reversible versus irreversible cell changes

Reversible cell injury or change – cell injury causes alteration or loss of cell function and structural changes, but the cell *can* recover and regain structure and function if the injuring stimulus is removed. These are also called *sublethal* cell injuries/changes.

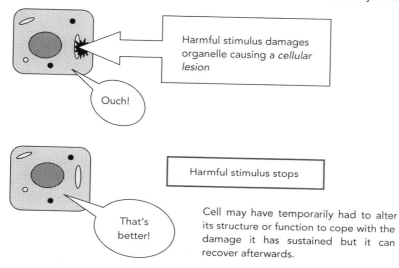

Harmful stimulus damages organelle causing a *cellular lesion*

Ouch!

Harmful stimulus stops

That's better!

Cell may have temporarily had to alter its structure or function to cope with the damage it has sustained but it can recover afterwards.

Irreversible cell injury – cell injury causes alteration or loss of cell function and structural changes, but the cell *cannot* recover if the stimulus stops or is removed. In other words, the cell passes a 'point of no return' and even if the harmful stimulus stops the cell will simply die (see *necrosis*).

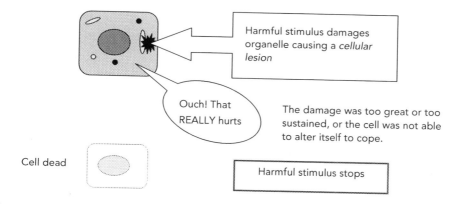

Harmful stimulus damages organelle causing a *cellular lesion*

Ouch! That REALLY hurts

The damage was too great or too sustained, or the cell was not able to alter itself to cope.

Cell dead

Harmful stimulus stops

Box 3.3 Factors affecting the type of cellular damage which occurs in response to a harmful stimulus

Factors specific to the injurious stimulus

- Duration – *how long the harmful stimulus goes on for*
- Size – *how large the harmful stimulus is*

Factors specific to the target tissue

- Blood supply – *how well supplied with blood the tissue is*
- Metabolic characteristics – *how metabolically active the tissue is*

broken down, but their constituents may not be entirely removed from the cytoplasm. They tend to accumulate as fatty, protein or crystal deposits and can often be seen when the cells are examined under the microscope.

- *Hydropic change* (cloudy swelling): Damage to cell membranes means that cells swell with fluid. Occurs in many cell types, e.g. early stages of liver cell damage by toxins.
- *Fatty change*: Fat (lipid) accumulates in cells because of increased or long-term fat breakdown in the body and thus the cells encounter increased or long-term levels of fat in their immediate environment. (This happens in malnutrition, when body fat is broken down and carried to the liver for metabolism, because there are inadequate dietary sources of energy. The liver cells therefore are presented with large amounts of fat in the blood entering the liver.) Fatty change can also occur because the ability of cells to metabolise *normal* amounts of fat is decreased by cell damage (decreased cell metabolism because of toxic damage, or reduced oxygen supply due to heart dysfunction, respiratory disease or anaemia, or in diabetes mellitus). Fatty change can be *idiopathic* (i.e. of uncertain cause) in the livers of older cats.
- *Pigments*: Accumulated pigments may be *endogenous* (produced by the body) such as haemosiderin (breakdown product of red blood cells, which may accumulate if there is marked red blood cell breakdown) or bile (again associated with breakdown of red blood cells). Bile pigments accumulate in disorders which cause jaundice, such as liver disease. Melanin is the brown pigment in skin and may accumulate in skin cells in certain conditions such as chronic dermatitis, causing the skin to darken.

  Accumulated pigments may also be *exogenous*, or foreign to the body, such as carbon from pollution, which may accumulate in the lungs of animals living in built-up areas. Other exogenous pigments can also accumulate in cells, indeed we make use of the fact since the inks used in tattoos accumulate in cells in the skin!

- *Proteins*: Viruses have to use cells of living creatures to manufacture protein as they do not have the capacity to do so for themselves; without using cells this way, viruses would not be able to reproduce themselves. Because of this, in some viral diseases, viral proteins accumulate within cells and can be seen under the microscope as so-called *viral inclusions*. Some viral inclusions are very characteristic in appearance and can help to make a diagnosis of a specific viral infection, even before virology has been carried out.

Box 3.4 Types of cellular degeneration

Cellular degenerations usually involve accumulation of substances within cells. There are various types of substances which may accumulate; this table is a summary of some of the more common intracellular accumulations.

In severe cases of the accumulation the affected organ will become swollen and discoloured.

Accumulation	Examples
- *Cellular components*	As cells age, old and non-functional organelles may shrivel up or be broken down, but their constituents may remain in the cytoplasm. They accumulate as fatty, protein or crystal deposits, and can be visible under the microscope.
- *Hydropic change* (cloudy swelling)	Damage to cell membranes means that cells swell with fluid, e.g. early stages of toxic damage to liver cells.
- *Fatty change*	Fat (lipid) accumulates in cells because of increased or long-term fat breakdown in the body (as in malnutrition) or because the ability of cells to metabolise *normal* amounts of fat is decreased by cell damage (e.g. decreased cell metabolism because of toxic damage or reduced oxygen supply or in diabetes mellitus). Fatty change can occur for uncertain reasons in the livers of older cats.
- *Pigments*	
○ *Endogenous*	Produced by the body, such as *haemosiderin* (from red blood cell breakdown), or *bile pigments* (accumulate in jaundice). *Melanin* accumulates in chronic dermatitis.
○ *Exogenous*	Foreign to the body, e.g. carbon from pollution, in the lungs of animals in built up areas, tattoo inks.
- Proteins	Accumulation of viral proteins within cells, can be seen microscopically as *viral inclusions*. Some viral inclusions are very characteristic and diagnostic.

Box 3.5 Common causes of necrosis

- Decreased blood supply (*ischaemia*, see Chapter 7) such as may occur when a blood vessel is damaged or blocked
- Pressure, for instance, from a tumour pressing on the area or prolonged presence of a tight bandage
- Burns – note that burns may be caused by heat, extreme cold (freezer burn) or caustic chemicals
- Trauma – causing damage to blood vessels or pressure on tissues
- Poisons and toxins – kill off cells by harmful effects on metabolism
- Infectious agents (*bacteria, viruses, fungi* and *parasites*) – damage cells in various ways

When the insult is severe or prolonged, the cell reaches a point at which it starts to die or undergo the process of necrosis, discussed next.

Cell death – necrosis

Necrosis is death of cells or tissues in a living animal. Note that when an animal dies the cells and tissues of that animal will also die as their oxygen supplies stop. This process is called *autolysis* and is not the same as necrosis, which is specifically death of cells in a living animal. There are a number of injurious stimuli that may result in necrosis (see Box 3.5). If you read through Box 3.5 you will see that these causes tend to involve either direct tissue damage *or* indirect damage due to injury to the blood supply of the tissue.

Not all necrosis in every tissue is the same in type or appearance. The type of necrosis that results in any given site depends on:

- the characteristics of the cells affected
- the characteristics of the tissues affected
- the cause of the necrosis
- other factors that might be involved, e.g. enzymes, bacteria and viruses

So, let us expand this list by discussing some different types of necrosis and their characteristic features.

Types of necrosis (see Boxes 3.6(a) and 3.6(b))

Coagulative necrosis
Coagulative necrosis is the most common type of necrosis and it occurs in many of the 'solid' organs such as the kidney and heart. Affected organs retain their structure and are pale and firm as though they had been cooked. The dead cells often retain their outline when viewed

under the microscope but are pale-staining and ghost-like. After a period of time, inflammatory cells move in to start to remove the dead cells (see Chapter 4), so the appearance of coagulative necrosis changes with time.

Proteins are released by the damaged and dying cells and are useful in the veterinary clinic as they can be detected in blood samples and used as diagnostic indications of the presence of tissue damage in certain organs. Examples of 'diagnostic' proteins are the enzymes creatine kinase (CK), increased plasma levels of which indicate muscle damage, and alanine aminotransferase (AAT) which are useful to indicate liver damage.

Liquefactive necrosis (sometimes called colliquative necrosis)

Liquefactive necrosis refers to areas of necrosis which become liquefied due to release of powerful enzymes which degrade the dead cells and extracellular components leaving a thick soup. This type of necrosis is characteristic after insults to the brain such as follows interruption of the blood supply (infarction, see Chapter 7) or bacterial infection (meningitis). In the latter case, the enzymes are produced by both the bacteria and by inflammatory cells which arrive to fight the infection. Liquefactive necrosis in the brain is also known as *malacia*.

Caseation necrosis

In caseation necrosis, the dead tissue is converted to a cream cheese texture (hence the name – caseous means 'cheesy'!). This type of necrosis is usually associated with chronic bacterial infections such as tuberculosis and is due to the presence of special fats in the bacterial wall which prevent liquefaction taking place.

Fat necrosis

Fat necrosis occurs after inflammation in/around fatty tissue, and occurs because enzymes degrade fat cells. The fat becomes hard and nodular. This is seen in the abdomen after pancreatitis, when pancreatic enzymes leak into the fat in the peritoneum. It can sometimes occur when fat in more peripheral areas is subjected to trauma and used to occur on the shoulders (withers) of draft animals, such as horses or oxen, with badly fitting harnesses.

Gangrene

Gangrene is a variant of coagulative necrosis and is the necrosis that occurs specifically due to loss of blood supply to an area, especially an extremity such as a foot, ear tip or tail. In most cases bacteria are involved and it is likely that the area was already contaminated with them when the necrosis was occurring. In all cases the affected part is cold to touch.

Four types of gangrene are described:

- *Dry gangrene*: No bacteria are involved. The tissue is dry and shrivelled, and is discoloured.
- *Gas gangrene*: Gas-producing bacteria proliferate in the necrotic tissue. The affected tissue has a crackly (*crepitant*) feel.
- *Moist gangrene*: Pus-producing bacteria proliferate in the areas of necrosis. This type of gangrene characteristically appears rotten and is very foul smelling (*putrefactive*).
- *Wet gangrene*: Bacteria are present and there is inflammation of adjacent non-necrotic tissue (inflammation in connective tissue is called *cellulitis*). The area swells and oozes fluid.

Sequelae of necrosis

'*Sequelae*' (plural), from '*sequel*' (singular) – in other words, what happens next, or the likely/possible next stages. The sequelae of necrosis depend on the tissue involved (such as its ability to regenerate its blood supply etc.), the extent of the necrosis and whether the injurious stimulus has stopped or whether it is ongoing.

Possible sequelae are listed below and some will be discussed further in the next few chapters. More than one of these possibilities may occur at any site of necrosis.

- *Tissue regeneration*: Healing of the area by replacement of dead cells by cells of the same type (see Chapter 6).
- *Scar formation*: Healing of the area by replacement of dead cells by fibrous (scar) tissue (see Chapter 6).
- *Erosion or Ulceration*: Loss of cells from a surface in or on the body, usually accompanied by inflammation (see Chapter 4). There is exposure of underlying tissues which is then vulnerable to bleeding (haemorrhage – see Chapter 7) or infection and continuation of inflammation.
- *Sequestration*: The area of dead and dying cells becomes walled-off (isolated) from the rest of the body by a dense rim of fibrous tissue, which means that the necrotic process, usually accompanied by inflammation (see Chapter 4), can continue inside (as an abscess). Sometimes the contents of the abscess break through the fibrous wall, spreading the inflammation and/or infection.

The preceding pages have discussed cellular changes in response to harmful stimuli. There are some changes which can occur outside or around cells (*extracellular changes*), and these are discussed below.

Box 3.6 (a) Types of necrosis

- *Coagulative necrosis*

    The most common type of necrosis, occurring in many of the 'solid' organs (e.g. kidney and heart).

    Affected organs retain their structure but are pale and firm (as though cooked). The dead cells retain their outline but are pale and ghost-like.

    After a period of time inflammatory cells move in to start to remove the dead cells (see Chapter 4), so the appearance of coagulative necrosis changes with time.

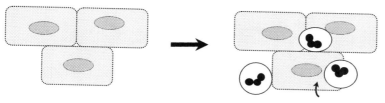

Inflammatory cell

Pale ghost-like cells retain their cellular outlines.

Eventually, the dead cells are removed by inflammatory cells.

- *Liquefactive necrosis* (sometimes called colliquative necrosis)

    Areas of necrosis which become liquefied by powerful enzymes which degrade the dead cells and surrounding tissues leaving a thick soup.

    Especially characteristic to the brain where it is called *malacia*, e.g. it occurs after interruption of the blood supply or bacterial infection (meningitis). In the latter case, the enzymes are produced by both the bacteria and by inflammatory cells which arrive to fight the infection.

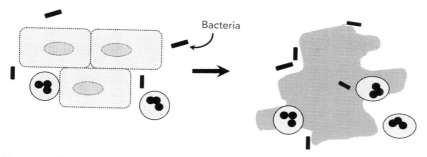

Bacteria

Necrotic cells and surrounding tissue liquefied by powerful enzymes produced by inflammatory cells and sometimes by bacteria.

Box 3.6 (a) (*Continued*) Types of necrosis

- *Caseation necrosis*

    The dead tissue is converted to a cheesy texture.

    Usually associated with chronic bacterial infections such as tuberculosis and is due to the presence of special fats in the bacterial wall which prevent liquefaction taking place.

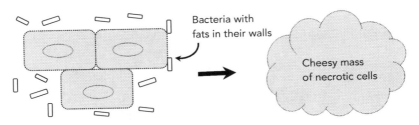

In certain chronic bacterial infections, such as tuberculosis, special fats in the bacterial wall prevent liquefaction of the necrotic tissue taking place. The dead tissue is converted to a cheesy texture.

- *Fat necrosis*

    Occurs after inflammation in/around fatty tissue, due to enzymes which degrade fat cells. The fat becomes hard and nodular.

    Seen after pancreatitis, when pancreatic enzymes leak into the abdomen. Sometimes occurs in fat subjected to trauma such as on the shoulders (withers) of draft animals, such as horses or oxen, with badly fitting harnesses.

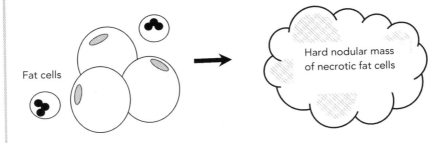

Inflammation in or around fatty tissue, with release of enzymes which then degrade fat cells. The fat becomes hard and nodular.

Box 3.6 (b) Summary of gangrene

- *Gangrene*

  A variant of coagulative necrosis.

  Occurs due to loss of blood supply to an area, especially extremities such as limbs, ears or tail tips.

  Bacteria are usually involved (contaminated wounds).

  In all cases the affected part is cold to touch.

Four types of gangrene described:
- *Dry* – no bacteria.

  The tissue is cold, shrivelled and discoloured.
- *Gas* – gas-producing bacteria proliferate.

  The affected tissue has a crackly feel (crepitus).
- *Moist* – pus-producing bacteria proliferate.

  Characteristically is rotten and foul smelling (putrefactive).
- *Wet* – bacteria are present and there is inflammation of adjacent non-necrotic tissue (*cellulitis*).

  The area swells and oozes fluid.

Extracellular changes (see Boxes 3.7 and 3.8)

Mineralisation

Calcification is the deposition of calcium salts in *normal* or *abnormal* tissues. Tissue containing deposited calcium salts is hard or gritty to touch and the calcium deposition can be felt as a scraping sensation when the tissue is incised with a knife. Two broad types are described – dystrophic calcification and metastatic calcification.

- *Dystrophic calcification*: In this form of calcification, calcium is deposited locally at sites *of tissue damage* (especially necrosis). For instance, it may occur in fatty tissue after pancreatic inflammation.
- *Metastatic calcification*: This form of calcification is associated with persistent high calcium levels throughout the body so that tissue is bathed in blood and fluids containing excess calcium. Causes of metastatic calcification include vitamin D toxicity, excess parathyroid hormone (or parathyroid-like hormone produced by certain tumours, see Chapter 8) and kidney failure.

Other examples of mineralisation
- *Dental plaque*: Gum inflammation, bacteria from the mouth and mineral in saliva combine to form a hard crust on the gums called plaque.

- *Kidney, bladder or bile stones* (*calculi*): The normal contents of a hollow or tubular organ become thickened by mucus or sediment; this, combined with bacteria, high local mineral levels and dead cells, allows formation of hard stones (calculi or liths). The stones vary slightly in colour and form depending on the mineral composition. See also urates/uric acid.

Crystals

Certain substances, entering via skin, lungs or intestinal tract, may lead to formation of crystalline material which can accumulate in various tissues. For instance, when animals drink liquid antifreeze (ethylene glycol) or eat certain plants, *calcium oxalate* crystals may accumulate in the kidneys (both inside and outside the cells) and cause necrosis and renal failure.

Urates/uric acid

Uric acid crystals and urates deposit in tissues in the disease called *gout*. This occurs when there is excess production or insufficient excretion of the metabolic waste-product uric acid. When uric acid levels in blood exceed a certain level, the uric acid can no longer remain dissolved in solution and urates or uric acid crystals deposit at various sites causing inflammation and pain. Gout occurs in the joints, kidneys and other organs (articular, renal and visceral forms of gout, respectively) in birds, snakes, mink and man.

Dogs normally convert uric acid to a protein (allantoin) in the liver as part of their metabolism. Dalmation dogs lack a liver enzyme required to metabolise uric acid in this way and consequently excrete uric acid in their urine. As a result, Dalmation dogs can develop urate or uric acid urinary calculi (uroliths).

Protein

A dense protein called *amyloid* can accumulate in certain chronic infectious, inflammatory, immune, metabolic or neoplastic diseases or as an aging change. Amyloid is an abnormal protein form, and, once produced and deposited, it is very resistant to removal by enzymes. As it builds up it can seriously hinder the function of affected tissues and even cause cell death.

Box 3.7 Summary of some of the main extracellular changes

Mineralisation	*Calcification (deposition of calcium salts in normal or abnormal tissues).*	• *Dystrophic calcification* – calcium is deposited *in areas of tissue damage* (especially necrosis), e.g. in fatty tissue after pancreatitis.
		• *Metastatic calcification* is associated with *persistent high body calcium levels* in blood and fluids, e.g. vitamin D toxicity, excess parathyroid hormone (or parathyroid-like hormone produced by certain tumours) and renal failure.

Dental plaque: Gum inflammation, bacteria and mineral in saliva combine to form a hard crust on the gums.

Kidney, bladder or bile stones (calculi): Contents of hollow or tubular organs can become thickened by mucus or sediment. When combined with bacteria, high mineral levels and dead cells hard calculi (or liths) may form.

Crystals   *Calcium oxalate* crystals can accumulate in the kidneys (both inside and outside the cells) and cause necrosis and renal failure. This occurs when animals drink liquid antifreeze (ethylene glycol) or eat certain plants.

Urates/uric acid

- *Gout* – deposition of uric acid crystals and urates in tissues. Occurs when there is excess production, or insufficient excretion, of the metabolic waste-product uric acid.

  Gout occurs in articular, renal and visceral forms in birds, snakes, mink and man.
- Dalmation dogs lack a liver enzyme required to metabolise uric acid to a protein (allantoin) in the liver, and excrete uric acid in their urine. Hence these dogs may develop urate or uric acid urinary calculi (uroliths).

Protein   A protein called *amyloid* can accumulate in certain chronic infectious, inflammatory, immune, metabolic or neoplastic diseases or as an aging change.

Amyloid is an abnormal form of protein, and it is very resistant to removal by enzymes. As it accumulates it can seriously hinder the function of affected tissues.

Box 3.8 Summary of cellular changes in response to a harmful stimulus discussed in Chapters 3 and 8

This table is intended as a checklist or a revision aid. You will need to get the details of each process from elsewhere in the book.

Reversible   *Cell degenerations* – intracellular accumulation of substances (*Chapter 3*)

- Old cellular components   Aging process
- Fluid   Hydropic change
- Lipids   Fatty change
- Proteins   Viral inclusions
- Pigments
  - endogenous   Bile pigment (bilirubin), haemosiderin, melanin
  - exogenous   Carbon, tattooing ink

Alterations of cell growth, size and number (see Chapter 8)

- Atrophy
- Hyperplasia
- Hypertrophy
- Metaplasia

Irreversible   *Cell death* – necrosis (*Chapter 3*)

- Coagulation
- Liquefaction
- Caseation
- Fat necrosis
- Gangrene
  - dry
  - gas
  - moist
  - wet

Alterations of cell growth, size and number (see Chapter 8)

- Neoplasia

Extracellular accumulations (*Chapter 3*)
- Mineral
  - dystrophic calcification
  - metastatic calcification
  - other   Dental plaque
- Crystals   Kidney, urinary bladder and gallstones
                                  Gout, calcium oxalate
- Protein   crystals
                                  Amyloid

Summary of key points in Chapter 3

- Gross pathological lesions are manifestations of changes/injury at cellular level.
- Cell changes can be reversible (the cell can recover when the harmful stimulus stops) or irreversible (cell dies or cannot return to normal) depending on factors specific to the harmful stimulus and to the tissue affected.
- Many reversible cell changes involve accumulation of endogenous or exogenous substances within the cell.
- Necrosis is an irreversible change. Types of necrosis vary according to the tissue affected and other factors involved.
- There are also extracellular accumulations or changes.

Test yourself questions on Chapter 3

1. Write short notes to define and illustrate the term 'lesion', including reference to reversible and irreversible cell changes.
2. Give three examples of types of cellular degeneration and associated clinical signs or conditions.
3. What is meant by the term *coagulative necrosis*? What does a tissue that has undergone coagulative necrosis look like? How may we detect necrosis in veterinary practice?
4. Tissue regeneration is one sequel of necrosis, name one other recognised sequel of necrosis.
5. Calcification is a common extracellular tissue degeneration.
   a. Define calcification and describe the physical appearance of calcified tissues.
   b. What is meant by dystrophic calcification?
   c. What is meant by metastatic calcification?
6. Gout occurs in certain veterinary species. What species are most at risk? What forms of gout are recognised? Briefly describe how gout is caused.

Chapter 4

Inflammation

What is inflammation?

Nomenclature

Acute inflammation

Chronic inflammation

Aims of Chapter 4

- To introduce the concept of inflammation as a protective response
- To become familiar with the vascular changes in acute inflammation, also the cells involved and the main histological features of acute and chronic inflammation
- To discuss local and systemic effects, potential harmful effects and sequelae of acute and chronic inflammation

What is inflammation?

Inflammation is a term used regularly in the clinical setting. Owners and veterinary professionals alike will say a particular area of skin, an eye or ear of an animal looks 'inflamed', but what do we mean when we say this? Usually, we are referring to redness, swelling and tenderness of the affected part; in this chapter, we will discuss what causes these grossly visible signs and the other less apparent components of inflammation.

Inflammation is defined as a *complex progression of blood vascular and tissue changes* that develops in response to tissue injury. What is often not appreciated is that inflammation is primarily a *protective response*. There are various protective mechanisms (phagocytic cells, leucocytes and antibodies) which circulate in the blood. Inflammation is a response that extends these defences of the blood out into the tissues, and prepares the way for repair of the tissue. The inflammatory response often works in concert with, and is directed by, cells of the immune system.

Whilst the *protective* role of inflammation is less commonly appreciated, the fact that uncontrolled or inappropriate inflammation can be harmful or destructive (even life-threatening if severe) is more commonly recognised. Inflammation which has become severe is usually the reason for animals with inflammatory conditions being presented at veterinary clinics for treatment. In veterinary species, inflammation is often exacerbated by self-harm (*self-trauma*) – scratching, licking, biting etc. – which can cause further tissue damage or introduce infection.

Inflammation is described as acute or chronic, and this infers not just the duration of the inflammatory response but also indicates differences in the inflammatory cells involved.

Nomenclature

We indicate inflammation in various organs or tissues by using the suffix (word ending) '-itis' after the Greek word for the organ. So, for instance,

Box 4.1 Summary of the introduction to inflammation

Inflammation is:

- usually denoted by *the suffix 'itis'* after the Greek word for the organ (e.g. hepatitis, nephritis, enteritis etc.)
- a complex *progression* of blood vascular and tissue changes that develops in response to tissue injury
- a *protective* response, which extends the defences of the blood out into the tissues and prepares the area for repair
- may become *uncontrolled or inappropriate*, and then can be painful, harmful or even life-threatening
- often exacerbated in veterinary species by *self-trauma* (scratching, licking and biting)
- described as *acute or chronic*, depending on the duration and cell types involved

inflammation in the liver is known as hepatitis; kidney, nephritis; small intestine, enteritis; colon, colitis; skin, dermatitis and so on.

See Box 4.1 for a summary of general information on inflammation.

So, let us consider the two types of inflammation – acute and chronic – in more detail, and discuss what these terms mean, and the differences between them.

Acute inflammation

From: *Latin 'acutus' = sharp*. Indicating a disease of *short and sharp course*

Acute inflammation is the initial reaction of a tissue to injury. It aims to rapidly contain, dilute and remove the harmful stimulus which has set off the inflammatory response, and to prepare the tissues for repair.

The (local) clinical signs of acute inflammation

There are five typical local signs of inflammation, which are also known as the *cardinal signs* of inflammation. These cardinal signs will be familiar to anyone who has seen an inflamed lesion. The cardinal signs are redness, heat in the tissue, pain and swelling, and often, loss of function of the affected part. Box 4.2 lists these cardinal signs again and in this box, next to each English term you will see a Latin term in italics. In some pathology textbooks you will see these Latin words used, as these are the terms coined by early pathologists, such as Celsus and Galen, who originally defined the cardinal signs of inflammation. Notice that the Latin term *tumor* is used but that this is a non-specific word for 'swelling' whereas we tend often to use it to mean a cancer or neoplastic growth (see further discussion of this in Chapter 8).

Box 4.2 The cardinal signs of acute inflammation

- Redness – *rubor*
- Heat – *calor*
- Pain – *dolor*
- Swelling – *tumor*
- Loss of function – *functio laesa*

Some pathology textbooks tend to use the Latin terms for each of these signs so these are included next to each English term in the list above. These Latin words are the terms coined by early pathologists who first defined these cardinal signs of inflammation.

   Notice that the Latin term *tumor* is used for swelling but that this term is often used to denote cancer or neoplastic growth (see further discussion of terminology of neoplasms in Chapter 8).

What causes acute inflammation? In other words, what do we mean by *harmful stimuli* for inflammation? There are a number of causes of inflammation such as presence of infectious agents or physical insults like trauma and burns. The immune system is involved in inflammation; indeed, the immune system is important in directing the inflammatory response. The immune system is also involved in inflammatory responses when it overreacts or reacts inappropriately to something (see Chapter 5). Finally, the presence of dead tissues (necrosis) for whatever reason, e.g. an interruption to the blood supply (see Chapter 7), can be a stimulus for an inflammatory response.

   Causes of acute inflammation include:

- Infection – *bacteria, fungi, viruses* and *parasites*
- Immune responses, hypersensitivities
- Physical causes – *trauma, heat, cold, radiation and chemicals*
- Presence of dead tissue (*necrosis*) due to a number of causes, e.g. *ischaemia* (see Chapter 7), or damaging effects of infectious organisms on cells

The three phases of acute inflammation

Acute inflammation is composed of three phases, which can be summarised as:

- *Vascular* – change in blood vessel diameter
- *Exudative* – increases in blood vessel leakiness resulting in fluid leakage from the circulation
- *Cellular* – leucocytes leave blood vessels, travel to site of injury and become activated

Box 4.3 Diagram of a capillary bed

Before considering the three phases of acute inflammation it is probably a good idea to remind ourselves that all tissues have a vast meshwork of fine blood vessels called capillaries (which form the *capillary bed*) and which receive arterial blood from the heart via an arteriole, and drain blood into the venous circulation, which carries it back to the heart. We will return to the capillary beds later (see Chapter 7), but here we are concerned particularly with their involvement in acute inflammation.

   Note the round cells, called mast cells, which are numerous in connective tissues – especially associated with blood vessels. We shall discuss mast cells and their actions in relation to phase 2 of acute inflammation.

Capillary bed in tissues

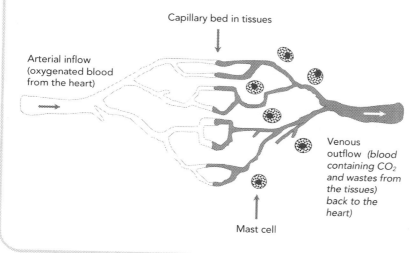

Arterial inflow (oxygenated blood from the heart)

Venous outflow *(blood containing CO$_2$ and wastes from the tissues) back to the heart)*

Mast cell

These three phases are discussed in more detail below. Note that during inflammation there will be overlap of the phases, and more than one phase may be occurring at any one time.

   Before considering the phases of acute inflammation it will be helpful to remember that all tissues have a meshwork of fine blood vessels (the *capillary bed*) which receives arterial blood from the heart via an arteriole, and drains blood into the venous circulation, which takes it back to the heart and then to the lungs. (See Box 4.3; see also Chapter 7 for more features of the circulatory system and capillaries in particular.)

Vascular phase of acute inflammation

The vascular phase is sub-divided into two parts:

1. *'White line'* is transient (lasting only a few seconds) and comprises a short period of constriction in the arteriole supplying

the capillary bed. The white line is a reflex smooth muscle response; you can demonstrate this by firmly dragging the blunt end of a pen across your skin. You should see a brief white line appear!

2. *Hyperaemia* is a longer period (lasting several minutes or even days) of arteriole and capillary dilation. This is caused by chemical mediators from the damaged tissue and from the plasma. Hyperaemia causes the area to become red and to feel warm (see Box 4.4). (Note that in American texts the spelling is *hyperemia*.)

Exudative phase of acute inflammation

The result of the exudative phase is, as the name suggests, escape or *exudation* of protein-rich fluid from the blood into the surrounding damaged tissue.

Exudation may be the result of direct damage to the lining (*endothelial*) cells of the capillaries since these endothelial cells can be injured by the same harmful stimulus that triggered the inflammatory response in the first place. Hence, physical damage, toxic agents, infection, enzymes and *oxygen free radicals* could stimulate exudation of fluid from blood into tissue. The injury to the endothelial cells simply makes them less efficient at lining blood vessels and the capillaries become leaky (at least, more leaky than normal – see Chapter 7). In the exudative phase of acute inflammation, however, we are really concerned with a 'deliberate' leakiness, orchestrated by cells of the acute inflammatory response. The chief cells involved in this are *mast cells*.

Mast cells are large round cells that are widespread in the body in connective tissues, strategically placed beside capillary beds (we introduced them in Box 4.3). Mast cells contain packets of potent chemicals in their cytoplasm (these packets are called *intracytoplasmic granules*). When mast cells are stimulated they release the contents of their intracytoplasmic granules (*degranulate*) so that the contents escape and act on nearby cells or tissues. The contents of mast cell intracytoplasmic granules include *histamine*, which has a number of biological effects, but importantly for our current discussion, histamine causes increased vascular *permeability* by stimulating the endothelial cells to contract. This cell contraction opens up holes in the capillary walls (*intercellular junctions*) allowing the escape of the protein-rich exudate into the surrounding tissue. Histamine is also, incidentally, able to cause vasodilation.

Mast cells can be triggered to degranulate by a number of stimuli and are not always acting in a protective way (see Box 4.5). It is the histamine from inappropriately stimulated mast cells that make hay fever sufferers' lives a misery at certain times of the year!

Box 4.4 Hyperaemia

Hyperaemia is part of the second phase of acute inflammation and consists of a period of arteriole and capillary dilatation, which can last for several minutes (or even days). This dilation of the vessels is caused by chemical mediators, such as those released by the damaged tissue.

Blood flow to the area markedly increases as a result of the vascular dilatation and this causes the area to become red and to feel warm (two of the cardinal signs of acute inflammation).

Normal capillary bed

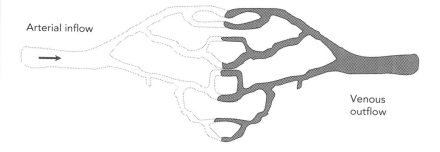

Arterial inflow

Venous outflow

Hyperaemic capillary bed in acute inflammation

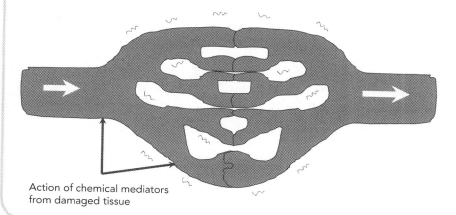

Action of chemical mediators from damaged tissue

Box 4.5 Mast cells and exudation

All blood vessels are lined by a layer of slender cells called *endothelial cells* which together make up the inner layer of the vessel wall – the *endothelium*. We will discuss the structure of capillaries more in Chapter 7; for now, it is the role of the endothelium in the exudative phase of acute inflammation which interests us.

Capillaries do not have much structure to their walls, so in effect the walls of capillaries are little more than a thin 'crazy paving' of endothelial cells (see diagram below). As a result they are naturally slightly leaky to fluid (see Chapter 7).

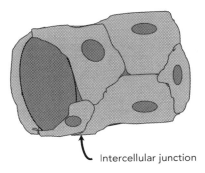

Intercellular junction

Diagram of a capillary – the wall is composed of a single layer of endothelial cells.

In the exudative phase of acute inflammation, we are really concerned with a 'deliberate' leakiness, orchestrated by cells of the acute inflammatory response. The chief cells involved in this process are *mast cells*.

Mast cells are large rounded cells that are widespread in the body in connective tissues, and especially in connective tissue surrounding capillary beds (see Box 4.3). Mast cells contain packets (called *intracytoplasmic granules*) of potent chemicals. When mast cells are stimulated (by various stimuli) they release the contents of their intracytoplasmic granules (a process called *degranulation*) so that the chemicals escape and can then act on nearby cells or tissues.

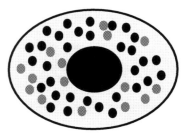

Diagram of a mast cell – the cytoplasm contains numerous granules which contain potent chemicals, such as histamine. When mast cells are stimulated to degranulate, the chemicals are released into the surrounding tissues.

The chemical contents of mast cell granules include *histamine* which has a number of biological effects including the ability to increase vascular *permeability* (leakiness) by stimulating the endothelial cells to contract. This cell contraction opens up gaps

Box 4.5 (*Continued*) Mast cells and exudation

between the endothelial cells (*intercellular junctions*) effectively forming holes in the capillary walls, and allowing the escape of the protein-rich fluid (*exudate*) into the surrounding tissue. Histamine is also able to cause vasodilation directly so can also contribute to the *vascular* phase of inflammation.

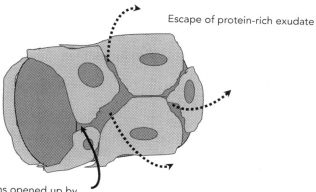

Escape of protein-rich exudate

Intercellular junctions opened up by the contraction of endothelial cells due to the effects of histamine

Mast cells respond to a number of triggers, and do not always have protective intentions. It is the effects of histamine from *inappropriately* stimulated mast cells that makes hay fever sufferers' lives such a misery at certain times of the year!

Note that exudation may also occur when there has been direct damage to the endothelial cells of the capillaries. These cells can be injured by the same harmful stimulus that triggered the inflammatory response in the first place. Hence, physical damage, toxic agents, infection, enzymes and *oxygen free radicals* can all stimulate exudation of fluid from blood into the tissues. The injury to the endothelial cells makes them less efficient at lining blood vessels and the capillaries become more leaky than normal, and more fluid leaks out than the drainage function of the venous and lymphatic circulations can cope with (see Chapter 7).

The leaked fluid accumulates in the tissues causing heat, swelling and pain (more cardinal signs of acute inflammation!)

Because the capillaries are made leaky by the opening up of gaps between the endothelial cells, large molecules in the blood (like proteins) and cells are also able to escape into the tissues. This is why inflammatory exudate is rich in protein. Normally, the proteins and cells are too large to pass through the intercellular junctions in the capillary walls. The typical composition of inflammatory exudate is shown in Box 4.6. Exudation of fluid causes swelling, heat and pain in the area.

Box 4.6 Typical contents of inflammatory exudate

Water
Electrolytes
Plasma proteins (*albumin*, *globulin* and *fibrinogen*)
Red blood cells
Platelets

Cellular phase of acute inflammation

The cellular phase of acute inflammation is a period of 'recruitment' of white blood cells (*leucocytes*) to the site of injury. The leucocytes aim to destroy bacteria at the site, to direct other cells of the inflammatory process and to start to clean up the mess by removing dead and dying cells, paving the way for the healing process to start.

The main leucocyte involved in acute inflammation is the neutrophil. See Box 4.7 for the main features of neutrophils.

Recruitment of neutrophils in the cellular phase of acute inflammation

In small veins (venules) and capillaries near the site of tissue damage, neutrophils *marginate*, which means they move towards the endothelial walls of the blood vessels, then they loosely stick to the walls and roll slowly along. At an intercellular junction between endothelial cells, they migrate out through the vessel wall (with the fluid exudate). Once in the tissue, using their natural motility, the neutrophils continue to migrate to the site of damage (see Box 4.8).

At the site of tissue damage the neutrophils degranulate, releasing their active granules into the area to kill bacteria (which they then ingest and destroy) and proteases to clean away the dead and dying tissue, thus preparing the site for healing (see Chapter 6).

When this cellular migration involves many cells, the fluid exudate which is also being produced becomes cloudy and is called a *cellular exudate*.

As well as local effects there are more general (*systemic*) effects of inflammation, discussed in the next section. You may recognise many of these as clinical signs in animals in your clinic.

Systemic effects of acute inflammation

- *Increased body temperature (fever)*
  - o Caused by chemical mediators of inflammation circulating in the blood and acting on temperature regulatory centres in the brain

Box 4.7 Essential features of the neutrophil

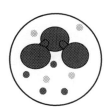 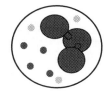

Cartoons of neutrophils. These small round cells have segmented nuclei and granules in their cytoplasm.

Features of neutrophils

- Neutrophils (NLs) are characteristic and diagnostic for acute inflammation
- NLs have segmented nuclei (see cartoons above)
- NLs have intracytoplasmic granules, the contents of which include
  ○ substances able to kill bacteria (*antimicrobial* factors)
  ○ enzymes able to digest protein (*proteases*)
- NLs originate in the bone marrow and circulate in the blood
- They do not live very long and if they attack bacteria they usually die in the process

Actions of neutrophils

- NLs are the first defence against invading microbes
- They are also involved in the initial removal of dead tissues
- They are able to move (*motile*), and are attracted to sites of tissue damage by chemical mediators produced by other cells
- NLs themselves produce mediators which regulate inflammation
- NLs stick to, ingest and destroy microbes by digesting them using the contents of their granules (*phagocytosis*) (see also macrophages, Box 4.12 – later this chapter)

- *Changes in blood (haematology)*
  ○ Increased release of *mature* neutrophils from bone marrow
  ○ Stimulation of production of new (*immature*) neutrophils – referred to as a '*shift to the left*' or a '*left shift*'
  ○ Possibly *anaemia* – the chemical mediators of inflammation can exert an inhibitory effect on the red cell producing part of bone marrow
- *Pain*
  ○ Direct nerve stimulation by chemical mediators or contents of neutrophil granules
  ○ Indirect due to fluid accumulation, forcing tissue components apart

Box 4.8 Recruitment of leucocytes in the cellular stage of acute inflammation

A: In venules and capillaries, the leucocytes (such as neutrophils or NLs) *marginate*, that is they move to the edge of the blood vessels and loosely stick to the endothelial wall. They then roll slowly along the walls.

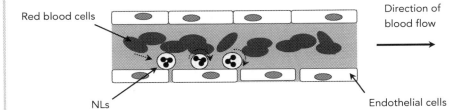

Red blood cells

Direction of blood flow

NLs

Endothelial cells

B: Near to the site of tissue damage, the leucocytes stop and squeeze through a junction between the endothelial cells.

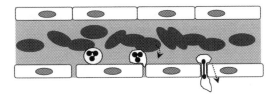

C: The leucocytes travel through the tissue until they reach the site of damage and then they release the contents of their granules (*degranulate*).

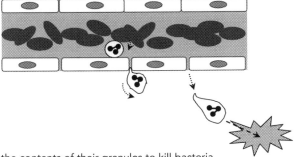

Leukocytes use the contents of their granules to kill bacteria, neutralise toxins, breakdown dead and dying tissue etc.

Site of tissue damage

- *Depression (malaise), anorexia, nausea*
  - Due to the effects of pain
  - Or due to the effects of chemical mediators on the brain
- *Muscle pain (myalgia)*
  - Breakdown of muscle by chemical mediators
- *Weight loss*
  - Muscle breakdown
  - Nausea, anorexia or pain causing loss of appetite
  - Or due to the effects of chemical mediators on appetite centres in the brain (Box 4.9)

Box 4.9 Systemic effects of acute inflammation

Increased body temperature (fever)	• Caused by chemical mediators of inflammation circulating in the blood and acting on temperature regulatory centres in the brain
Changes in haematology	• Increased release of *mature* neutrophils from bone marrow • Stimulation of production of new (*immature*) neutrophils – referred to as a '*shift to the left*' or '*left shift*' • Possibly *anaemia* – the chemical mediators of inflammation can exert an inhibitory effect on the red cell-producing part of bone marrow
Pain	• Direct nerve stimulation by chemical mediators or contents of neutrophil granules • Indirect due to fluid accumulation, forcing tissue apart
Depression (malaise), anorexia, nausea	• Due to the effects of pain • Or due to the effects of chemical mediators on the brain
Muscle pain (myalgia)	• Breakdown of muscle by chemical mediators
Weight loss	• Muscle breakdown • Nausea, anorexia or pain causing loss of appetite • Or due to the effects of chemical mediators on appetite centres in the brain

Some specific types of acute inflammation

The above description is a general account of acute inflammation, involving production of a cellular (neutrophilic) exudate. There are some specific types of acute inflammation, which involve different types of exudate. For instance:

- *Serous* exudate has a low cell content but is composed of the high protein fluid described earlier in this chapter.
- *Haemorrhagic* exudate contains numerous red blood cells in the serous fluid, with or without leucocytes.
- *Fibrinous* exudate contains abundant sticky protein called fibrin (see also discussion of blood clotting in Chapter 7). This type of exudate is often produced when serous membranes, such as the pleura or peritoneum are inflamed (see section *Harmful effects of acute inflammation*).
- *Purulent* or *suppurative* exudate contains many dead and dying neutrophils and bacteria (*pus*) (see section *Harmful effects of acute inflammation*).
- In addition to these, combinations may occur such as *mucopurulent* or *necrohaemorrhagic* exudates, but do not worry too much about these terms!

Remember, inflammation aims to protect the body by seeking out and destroying damaging or harmful stimuli (whatever they may be), limiting their spread and cleaning up afterwards so that healing can ensue. Sometimes, however, inflammation can have harmful effects on the animal and we have discussed some of these when looking at systemic effects of acute inflammation. The following list indicates some of the especially bad effects of acute inflammation.

Harmful effects of acute inflammation (see Box 4.10)

- *Excessive tissue damage*: Remember that leucocytes like neutrophils contain enzymes that digest proteins, and they do not care what proteins they digest. If lots of neutrophils are activated, there can therefore be damage to surrounding tissue, not just the site of the original damage.
- *Systemic effects may be severe*: If you refer again to the list of systemic effects of acute inflammation you will appreciate that in severe cases there is the potential for considerable pain, loss of appetite, weight loss and fever, for instance.
- *Excessive loss of serum*: This can cause marked swelling, with problems of pain, irritation and self-trauma. In really severe cases, fluid loss may contribute to shock (see Chapter 7).
- *Inflammation of vessel walls (vasculitis)*: Vasculitis can cause excessive leakiness of blood vessels, haemorrhage or tendency for blood

to clot inappropriately (*thrombosis*), and can impair blood supply to tissue (*ischaemia* and *infarction*) (see Chapter 7).

- *Hypersensitivity reactions*: In animals sensitive to certain protein triggers (*allergens*) mast cell degranulation can be excessive and the immune system can direct a very marked and inappropriate inflammatory response. Some of the very itchy skin diseases we see in veterinary species are examples of hypersensitivities; these conditions often involve eosinophils instead of neutrophils (see later).
- *Severe fibrin exudation*: As noted above, the sticky protein fibrin tends to accumulate on serous membranes such as *pleura* (which cover the lungs and line the rib cage), the *pericardium* (around the heart), or the *peritoneum* (which surrounds the abdominal contents). The fibrin subsequently is replaced by fibrous tissue (by the process of organisation – see Chapter 6) forming a firm scar (*adhesion*). In some circumstances and locations, this fibrous scarring can be damaging and hinder normal function of the organ. For instance, pleural adhesions that form after severe pneumonia can affect lung expansion. Adhesions forming after inflammation of peritoneum (*peritonitis*) may bind segments of gut tightly together or even encircle the gut causing an effective blockage of the intestine.
- *Suppurative exudate*: Suppurative exudate can become walled off by fibrous tissue and remain as a pocket of inflammation (called an *abscess*) which refuses to clear up or occasionally bursts out. Abscesses which choose to burst internally may lead to conditions such as septic peritonitis or pericarditis, which in worst cases may lead to potentially fatal septic shock (see Chapter 7).

Box 4.11 is a handy summary of acute inflammation. We now move on from acute inflammation to discuss longer-term inflammatory responses.

Chronic inflammation

From: *Greek 'chronos'* = *time, of long duration*; indicating a disease of *slow progress and long continuance*

Chronic inflammation is defined as the persistence of the inflammatory response for longer than approximately 10–14 days (perhaps up to year or more). Compare the time scale of acute inflammation earlier in this chapter.

Chronic inflammation is not exudative and involves the formation of fibrous tissue (*fibrosis*, see Chapter 6). Different cells are involved too, with *macrophages* (Box 4.12) and cells of the immune system (*lymphocytes* and *plasma cells*; Box 4.13) being important. Mast cells and neutrophils play lesser roles in chronic inflammation, if they are involved at all.

Box 4.10 Harmful effects of summary of acute inflammation

Excessive tissue damage	Leucocytes like NLs contain enzymes that digest proteins indiscriminately. If lots of NLs are activated they can damage surrounding tissue, not just the site of the original damage.
Systemic effects may be severe	In severe inflammation there may be considerable pain, loss of appetite, weight loss and fever.
Excessive loss of serum	Causes marked swelling, with pain, irritation and self-trauma. If very severe, fluid loss may contribute to shock.
Inflammation of vessel walls (vasculitis)	Causes excessive leakiness of blood vessels, and haemorrhage or inappropriate clotting (*thrombosis*), impairing blood supply to tissue (*ischaemia* and *infarction*).
Hypersensitivity reactions	In animals sensitive to certain protein triggers (*allergens*) mast cell degranulation can be excessive and the immune system directs a marked and inappropriate inflammatory response, e.g. very itchy skin diseases (often involving eosinophils instead of NLs).
Severe fibrin exudation	Fibrin accumulates on serous membranes, e.g. the *pleura, pericardium* or *peritoneum*. The fibrin is replaced by fibrous tissue (*organisation*) forming a scar (*adhesion*). In some circumstances and locations this fibrous scarring hinders normal function of the organ.
Suppurative exudate becomes walled off by fibrous tissue	Remains as an *abscess*, which refuses to clear up or bursts. Abscesses which burst internally may lead to septic peritonitis or pericarditis, which can cause potentially fatal septic shock.

Box 4.11 Summary of acute inflammation

Vascular – change in blood vessel diameter. White line followed by hyperaemia.
Exudative – increase in blood vessel leakiness resulting in fluid loss. Mast cells are important.
Cellular – leucocytes leave blood vessels, travel to site of injury and become activated (degranulate). NLs are important.

Box 4.12 Features of macrophages

Cartoon of a macrophage

A large rounded cell with a single rounded nucleus

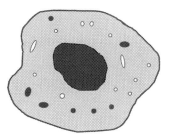

Features of macrophages

- Macrophages are large rounded cells with single rounded nuclei
- They are produced in the bone marrow
- They travel in the blood (as *monocytes*) and enter the tissue (and then are called macrophages) (see diagram below)
- They are longer-lived than NLs, with a 30–60 day life span
- They are larger and move more slowly than NLs

Origin of tissue macrophages

Monocyte in blood circulation

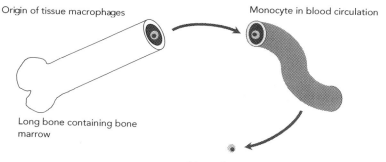

Long bone containing bone marrow

Macrophage in tissue

Actions of macrophages

- Very efficient at phagocytosis. Have intracytoplasmic vacuoles containing enzymes which they use to digest the target (see A. B. and C. below)
- Macrophages do not necessarily die when they attack a target and can live to fight another day (unlike NLs)
- They can digest a wider range of targets than NLs, including foreign material
- In the case of particularly persistent targets, foreign material that is hard to digest for instance, macrophages are directed by lymphocytes to increase their killing power by joining forces. When they do this they form very large cells with lots of nuclei (*multinucleated giant cells*) (see D. below)
- Macrophages also produce mediators which regulate inflammation, immune response, and repair processes

Box 4.12 (Continued) Features of macrophages

Phagocytosis

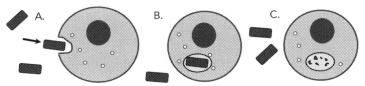

A. The macrophage engulfs a particle to be destroyed, keeping it in a vacuole within its cytoplasm. B. Enzymes from its intracytoplasmic granules are secreted into the vacuole. C. The particle is broken down and eventually the fragments may be extruded ("spat out") by the macrophage, which can then attack another foreign particle.

D.

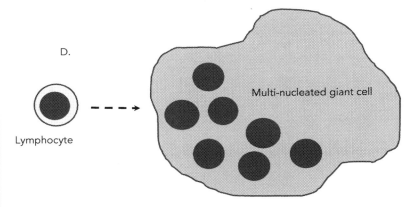

Multi-nucleated giant cell

Lymphocyte

With very persistent inflammatory stimuli (e.g. foreign material), macrophages may be directed by lymphocytes to gang together and form multi-nucleated giant cells.

Chronic inflammation is often also accompanied by reactive *hyperplasia* or *hypertrophy* in surrounding tissues (see Chapter 8), because the mediators which encourage fibrous tissue formation can stimulate division and growth of other cells too.

The main types of chronic inflammation

Two main types of chronic inflammatory response are described, known as *granulomatous* and *non-granulomatous* (or diffuse) chronic inflammation, which refers to the pattern of inflammatory cells seen under the microscope.

Box 4.13 Lymphocytes and plasma cells

A lymphocyte – a small round cell with sparse cytoplasm and a round nucleus.

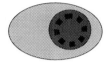

A plasma cell – a medium-sized oval cell with a round nucleus towards one end, which looks a bit like a clock face.

Features and actions of lymphocytes and plasma cells

- Lymphocytes are small and round with relatively little cytoplasm. Plasma cells are oval shaped. Both have round nuclei and are sometimes known as the *mononu-clear* cells
- They are of bone marrow or thymus origin
- They are important cells of the immune system
- They are involved when the immune system directs inflammatory processes
- Lymphocytes produce inflammatory mediators which regulate chronic inflammation
- Plasma cells are a variant of lymphocytes and produce *antibodies* (see Chapter 5)

Non-granulomatous chronic inflammation involves loose clusters of inflammatory cells with no particular arrangement and a variable background of fibrosis, or with reactive *hyperplasia* or *hypertrophy* in surrounding tissues (see Chapter 7). So, chronically inflamed skin may thicken and become greasy because of hyperplasia in the skin glands. The wall of chronically inflamed gut may also become thickened compared with normal.

Granulomatous chronic inflammation describes inflammation composed of distinct arrangements of inflammatory cells called *granulomas* (see Box 4.14). Granulomas are made up of central collections of macrophages with other mainly *mononuclear* inflammatory cells clustered around the macrophages and a rim of fibrous tissue around the outside.

Specialised forms of macrophages may be present, such as *multinucleated giant cells* (see Box 4.12) which are formed by fusion of macrophages. Some chronic inflammatory responses are called *pyogranulomatous*. This means that there are neutrophils as well as macrophages in the centre of the granulomas. Feline infectious

Box 4.14 Structure of a granuloma (*diagrammatic and not to scale*)

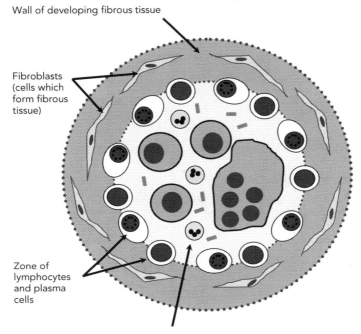

Wall of developing fibrous tissue

Fibroblasts (cells which form fibrous tissue)

Zone of lymphocytes and plasma cells

Central area contains:
- macrophages (and possibly multinucleated giant cells)
- there may also be neutrophils in certain circumstances (*pyogranulomatous* inflammation)
- dead and/or dying cells
- proteins
- foreign material or infectious agents

This diagram demonstrates the structure of granulomas in chronic granulomatous inflammation. The components of a granuloma tend to form recognisable patterns, so that macrophages (and neutrophils, if present) will be central, surrounded by a zone of lymphocytes and plasma cells, and all are encircled by variably mature fibrous tissue (depending how long-standing is the granuloma).

Granulomas may be single and large (grossly visible lumps) or they may be smaller and multiple so the affected tissue feels thickened and nodular (lumpy).

Granulomas form when the cause of the inflammation resists destruction by other inflammatory or immune-mediated processes. Foreign material (sutures or splinters) will stimulate a granulomatous inflammatory response, as will resistant infectious organisms, like bacteria with capsules of waxy coats (e.g. the tuberculosis bacillus) or parasites with tough outer walls.

Some immune responses are associated with granuloma formation and, in certain cases, hypersensitivities.

peritonitis (FIP) virus causes inflammation which is characteristically *pyogranulomatous* (see also Chapter 5).

Granulomas may be single and large (grossly visible lumps) or they may be smaller and there may be lots of them, so an affected tissue feels thickened and nodular (lumpy). They form when the cause of the inflammation resists destruction by other inflammatory or immune-mediated processes. Foreign material, like sutures or splinters, will initiate granulomatous inflammation, as will resistant infectious organisms, like bacteria with protective capsules or waxy coats (such as in tuberculosis) or parasites with tough outer walls. Certain immune responses are associated with granuloma formation and, in certain cases, hypersensitivities.

Eosinophilic granuloma in cats

A specific granulomatous condition, which does not involve the typical cell types discussed above, is eosinophilic granuloma complex (EGC) in cats. Eosinophilic granuloma is actually a hypersensitivity reaction; in other words, the cat's immune system is responding specifically, but inappropriately or in an exaggerated way, to a particular stimulus. EGC comprises a number of skin lesions, often involving the lip or face. The lesions are firm and usually ulcerated. Eosinophils have granules in their cytoplasm (*intracytoplasmic granules*), the contents of which are quite damaging to tissues (Box 4.15). Eosinophil accumulation and activation (*degranulation*) is usually accompanied by local tissue damage which stimulates a secondary acute inflammatory response.

Sometimes we do not know the stimulus for EGC (an *idiopathic* response), but one example of an eosinophilic granulomatous inflammatory response in cats occurs as a hypersensitivity reaction to an insect such as a mosquito, biting the cat on a sensitive area such as the nose.

Returning to the more typical manifestation of chronic inflammation, we now discuss what harmful effects it can have on the animal.

Harmful effects of chronic inflammation

- *Long-term diseases*: Chronic inflammation is often associated with long-term diseases, which result from lasting dysfunction of the affected organ or tissue. For instance, persistent renal disease due to chronic nephritis (inflammation of the kidney), or unremitting diarrhoea or weight loss due to chronic enteritis.
- *Weight loss or poor weight gain*: As well as possible direct effects of the chronic inflammatory process there can be weight loss or poor weight gain due to chronic effects of chemical mediators (see also *Systemic effects of acute inflammation*).

Box 4.15 Eosinophils

Features and actions of eosinophils

- Eosinophils (ELs) are formed in bone marrow
- Like neutrophils (NLs), they are small round cells with multilobed nuclei, but they stain a slightly different colour to NLs in histological sections – tending to look red
- Horse ELs are expanded by lots of large granules, which makes them look like small bunches of grapes under the microscope

                    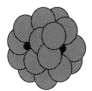

Eosinophil   Horse eosinophil

- ELs are less numerous in the blood than NLs, but are readily produced when needed
- ELs are motile (like NLs)
- They have intracytoplasmic granules which contain
  - Enzymes similar to NLs
  - Also, a range of additional highly active degradative and anti-inflammatory proteins specific to ELs
- ELs are associated with:
  - Parasite infestations
  - Allergic reactions and hypersensitivities
- ELs are phagocytic though less so than NLs. ELs tend to damage larger agents (like parasites) by releasing their granule contents towards the target. Other inflammatory cells can then move in to remove the remains of the target
- ELs can damage tissue if they over-secrete their enzymes (for instance in allergies)

- *Loss of organ/tissue function*: There can be loss of tissue function due to the presence of the inflammatory process, for instance, chronically inflamed gut will not absorb nutrients efficiently, but also chronic inflammation may cause unremitting pain, swelling, fibrosis (scar formation), discharge (if associated with a focus of walled-off suppuration) and so on. Muscles in affected limbs may atrophy, or scar tissue becomes excessive, or there may be metaplasia of epithelial cells to another type with different functions (see Chapter 8).

- *Tumour formation*: In rare cases, chronic inflammation may even lead to formation of a tumour at the site.
- *Recurrent or persistent fever*: It may occur due to persistent high levels of inflammatory mediators.
- *Changes in the blood*: Long-term stimulation of the bone marrow and utilisation of white cells can alter the haematology results. The white cells will tend to increase as will levels of proteins called *globulins* which are associated with antibodies (see Chapter 5), but there will usually be a decrease in the red cell producing part of the bone marrow, so chronic inflammation is accompanied by anaemia.

One final note on spelling, have you noticed that 'inflamed' contains only one 'm', whilst 'inflammation' has two of them? These are two more words that examiners like to see spelt correctly!

Summary of key points in Chapter 4

- Inflammation is a complex progression of vascular and cellular changes in response to tissue injury, which operates in concert with the immune system.
- Inflammation is a protective response, but sometimes it becomes exaggerated, inappropriate or harmful.
- Acute inflammation is the initial short-term response, in which blood vessels dilate and become permeable with escape of fluid exudate, and white blood cells such as neutrophils are recruited from the vessels.
- Chronic inflammation occurs in the presence of continued or longer term stimuli and is dominated by macrophages and cells of the immune system (lymphocytes and plasma cells) with fibrous tissue.
- Granulomas are a specific discrete pattern of chronic inflammation, though chronic inflammation can also be diffuse (non-granulomatous).

Test yourself questions on Chapter 4

1. Define the term 'inflammation' and then write some brief notes on the main features of inflammatory responses.
2. a. Name the three phases of acute inflammation.
   b. What are the five (local) clinical (or cardinal) signs of acute inflammation and what phase(s) of acute inflammation do you think are likely to contribute to each of the signs you have listed?
3. a. Why is the tissue fluid which results in the exudative phase of acute inflammation high in protein?
   b. List three typical components of an inflammatory exudate, apart from protein.
4. Describe how an abscess may form at the site of inflammation.
5. Briefly discuss the difference between acute and chronic inflammation, remembering to indicate which cells are important.
6. a. What are the two main types of chronic inflammation and briefly indicate the appearance of each of these types of chronic inflammatory response.
   b. Draw a simple diagram of a granuloma – indicate arrangement of the main cell types likely to be involved.
   c. Give an example of a veterinary disease characterised by granulomatous inflammation.

Chapter 5

Pathology and the Immune System

The normal immune system

Why do animals need an immune system?
How does the immune system work?
The lymphocyte families

Diseases of the immune system

Disorders of reduced immune function
Disorders of increased or inappropriate immunity

The normal immune system

Why do animals need an immune system?

Animals (and humans) encounter potentially harmful infectious agents all the time. On a daily basis, bacteria, viruses or fungal spores may be swallowed or inhaled, try to colonise the skin, urinary or reproductive tracts, or may penetrate the mucous membranes. Some form of defence system is vital for survival in the face of these potential invasions.

As humans we try to live as hygienically as possible to reduce our levels of exposure to infectious organisms; we try to keep ourselves and our environments as clean as we can. If we keep or care for animals, we clean them out regularly and ensure that they have clean water and fresh food. This care is even more important with sick humans or animals who are especially vulnerable to infections.

Whilst we can reduce our exposure to potential infections by hygiene we do not and cannot rely entirely on cleanliness to avoid infectious diseases. Fortunately, our bodies possess complex defences, called the *immune responses*, which serve to protect us from infections. In most cases, the immune system works well and infectious agents are immobilised or destroyed, and fail to cause clinical disease.

In this chapter, we will briefly review how the immune system normally works. The immune system is highly complex, however, and more detailed study of its function and role is beyond the scope of this book; you are advised to refer to the readings lists at the back of the book for suggestions of more comprehensive references if you need them.

Sometimes, the immune response is overwhelmed or is unable to work adequately, and we will discuss this when we look at diseases due to *immunodeficiency* or *immunosuppression*. We also need to consider diseases which occur when the immune system fails to distinguish between potentially harmful things and the body's own tissues, a phenomenon known as *autoimmunity*.

How does the immune system work?

The immune system is divided into two broad categories, *innate* and *adaptive* immunity.

Innate (natural or native) immunity

One of the first types of defence is known as the *innate* immune response (also sometimes called the *natural* or *native* immune system). Innate immunity is composed of chemical mediators of inflammation (see Chapter 4 for discussion of inflammation) and several plasma proteins, as well as cells able to phagocytose (ingest and destroy) foreign material, such as *neutrophils* and *macrophages*, and a specific type of *lymphocyte* with the heroic name of *natural killer* (NK) *cells* (see later note) (see Box 5.1).

In addition to components of the innate immune system, various natural barriers of the body act as physical barriers to invasion – the fortress walls. These barriers include the epithelial covering surfaces of structures such as the skin, respiratory or urinary tracts or gut. In some areas, the epithelial surfaces are further protected by mucus, fats (such as sebum on the skin's surface) or protein (such as the top – *cornified* – surface of the skin), or by the tiny hair-like structures called cilia, which help to clear mucus and foreign material out of the respiratory tract.

Physical barriers and the innate immune responses are the first lines of defence that protect us from the majority of infections that continually challenge us. The innate immunity is able to respond very rapidly, within hours, of an encounter with an infectious agent. It recognises broad groupings of foreign molecules (known as *antigens* – see later). In other words, the innate immune response recognises 'families' of bacteria and viruses, though does not act specifically towards individual members of the families as does the adaptive immune response, discussed next.

Adaptive (acquired or specific) immunity

The other broad category of the immune response is known as *adaptive* immunity (also known as *acquired* or *specific* immunity). Adaptive immunity is formed by mechanisms that are stimulated to respond by *specific* infectious agents, but which can also recognise and react to lots of other foreign molecules. Another characteristic of the adaptive immune response is that it develops a 'memory' of the required response for a particular foreign molecule. Next time the animal encounters a similar infection, the immune response to that particular infectious agent can be 'recalled' – this is also important in the response to vaccines and will be discussed again later.

Before we continue it would be worth defining a word which will crop up many times during our discussion of the adaptive immune system –

Box 5.1 Diagram of the components of innate immunity

The innate immune system (also called the *natural* or *native* immune system) is the body's first line of defence. It is always ready to act to prevent invasion by infectious agents. The innate immune responses are able to respond very rapidly (within hours) of encountering an infectious agent. They recognise broad 'families' of bacteria and viruses, though its response is not as specific as that of the adaptive immune response.

The innate immune response includes chemical mediators of inflammation (*cytokines*) and several plasma proteins as well as cells able to phagocytose (ingest and destroy) foreign material, such as *neutrophils* and *macrophages*, and a specific type of *lymphocyte* called a *natural killer cell*.

As well as the cells, proteins and chemical messengers of innate immunity, the body's first defences to invasion include physical barriers such as epithelial surfaces of skin, respiratory or urinary tracts or gut and other protective devices such as cilia, mucus, fats or protein layers.

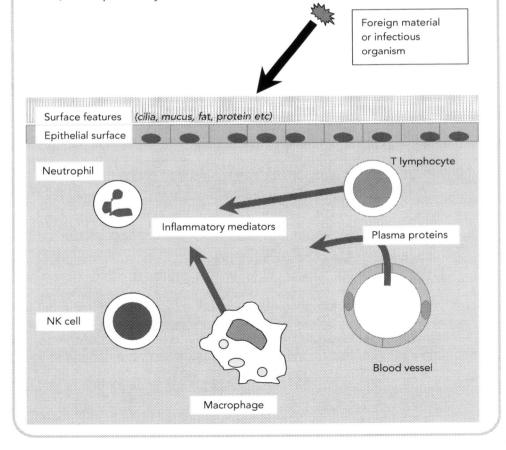

antigen. Antigen comes from the term *antibody-generating*, referring to a molecule able to stimulate the production of specific antibodies as part of the immune response. A molecule which can stimulate antibody production in this way is also said to be *antigenic*. As you will see later, we now know that the immune system involves more than antibodies, so the modern definition implies all substances that are recognised by, and stimulate a response in, the adaptive immune system. The word *immunogen* may also be used for this property, and such a molecule is then said to be *immunogenic*. But do not worry too much about the distinction between these terms at this stage.

Antigens are usually proteins or complex sugars which are part of bacteria, viruses and other microorganisms. Thus, not only parts of the microorganism's capsule or cell wall, or the flagellae (tendrils which help the organism move), but also toxins produced by the organism, may be antigenic. Host cells may also carry an antigenic molecule on their cell membranes, if they are infected with a virus or have *phago-cytosed* an infectious organism.

Some molecules which are not produced by microbes, such as pollens, may also be antigenic since the immune system recognises them as foreign to the body (non-'self'). Tumour cells are sometimes so abnormal that they too can carry surface markers which are antigenic to the host's own immune system. Other clinically significant examples of non-microbial antigens are proteins associated with transplanted tissue cells or transfused blood cells since these can stimulate an immune response in the recipient animal, causing rejection of tissue transplants or widespread destruction of transfused blood cells leading to anaemia and jaundice.

At this stage, it is worth making sure that you are familiar with the main cell types involved in the adaptive immune system, which are *lymphocytes*, *plasma cells* and *macrophages*. We met these cells in the previous chapter when we discussed inflammation. Try the test yourself questions in Box 5.3 and refer back to Chapter 4 for more details, before you read on.

You should have noticed that macrophages appear in both the descriptions of the *innate* and *adaptive* immunity. We will come back to this later.

The following is a simplified discussion of the adaptive immune system. As previously suggested, if you need more details on immunology you are recommended to have a look at one of the excellent books on veterinary immunology (some are suggested in the section of further reading at the end of this book).

Note from Box 5.2 that the main cells of the immune system belong to certain cell families. It is easiest to consider these families in turn as we discuss the immune response.

Box 5.2 Diagram of cells of the adaptive immune response (see text for more details)

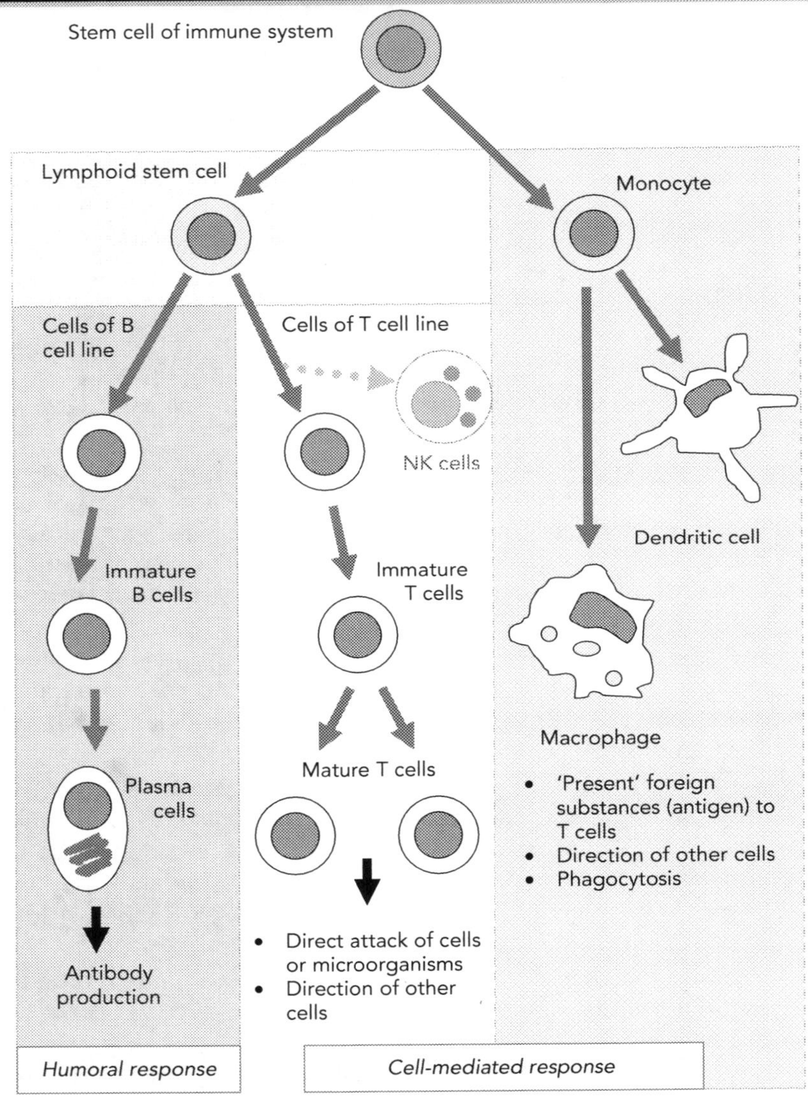

Stem cell of immune system

Lymphoid stem cell

Monocyte

Cells of B cell line

Cells of T cell line

NK cells

Dendritic cell

Immature B cells

Immature T cells

Mature T cells

Macrophage

Plasma cells

- 'Present' foreign substances (antigen) to T cells
- Direction of other cells
- Phagocytosis

Antibody production

- Direct attack of cells or microorganisms
- Direction of other cells

Humoral response

Cell-mediated response

Box 5.3 Test yourself revision box on macrophages, lymphocytes and plasma cells (see Chapter 4 for more details on these cells)

1. What do macrophages look like? – i.e. are they large or small cells? How many nuclei do they have? What shape are their nuclei?

    ....

    ....

    ....

2. Where in the body are macrophages produced?

    ....

3. Macrophages travel from their site of origin in the blood to the tissues. What are they called when they are in the blood?

    ....

4. Macrophages are very efficient at phagocytosis. What is meant by phagocytosis? Name another phagocytic cell type.

    ....

5. With what type of inflammation are macrophages especially associated?

    ....

    ....

6. Lymphocytes and plasma cells are sometimes called the mononuclear cells. What do lymphocytes look like?

    ....

    ....

7. How do plasma cells differ in appearance from lymphocytes?

    ....

8. What are the sites of origin of lymphocytes and plasma cells?

    ....

    ....

9. Lymphocytes are involved when the immune system and inflammation are linked. How do lymphocytes regulate inflammation?

    ....

    ....

10. What important part of the immune response do plasma cells produce?

    ....

    ....

The lymphocyte families

Lymphocytes are small round cells with sparse cytoplasm and single round nuclei. Lymphocytes are found throughout the body tissues and in the blood and lymph, but they are especially associated with organs of the lymphoid system (such as the lymph nodes, bone marrow, spleen and the thymus in young animals). Lymphocytic cells belong to the B cell line or the T cell line; each line has different specific roles in the immune response.

The B cell line

Lymphocytes of the B cell line (known as B cells) originate in the bone marrow in mammals and are found in lymph nodes, the spleen and in bone marrow, where their major role is production of antibodies as part of the immune response.

Antibodies (also known as immunoglobulins or Igs)

These are specialised proteins which recognise and help to destroy foreign material (antigen – discussed earlier), including infectious agents such as bacteria and viruses. Antibodies are formed from paired chains of proteins of different sizes (known as heavy and light chains), which are linked so that the structure forms a sort of 'Y' shape (see Box 5.4).

In mammals there are five different groups of antibody, known as *isotypes*, which are classified according to the type of heavy chain they have. Each of the groups performs different roles in the body, and helps the immune system to make the appropriate response to each type of 'foreign' object the body encounters.

Although the general structure of all antibodies is similar, a region at the very tip of the arms of the 'Y' shape is very variable. This variability of the tip structure means that millions of antibodies with slightly different structures exist. It is this variable region that recognises and binds to a distinct part of an antigen in a highly specific way, like a unique key which fits only one lock. The antigen-binding site is actually formed by the cleft between the tip of a light chain and a heavy one (refer again to Box 5.4). This highly specific binding allows antibodies to identify and attach only to their target antigen – in the midst of the millions of different molecules which they may encounter – both foreign and 'self' (see later, this section).

The many variants of antibody, each able to bind to a different target, allow for a huge diversity of antibodies and means that the immune system is able to recognise an enormous range of different antigens.

When an antibody recognises and attaches to an antigen it effectively 'labels' the antigen, marking it out for attack by other parts of the immune system. Antibodies can also directly inhibit the harmful effects of an infectious agent by, for example, binding to and

Box 5.4 (a) Diagram of an antibody (immunoglobulin). (b) Diagrammatic representation of an immunoglobulin on the surface of a B cell, acting as an antigen receptor for the cell

Antibodies (immunoglobulins) are formed from paired chains of proteins of different sizes (known as heavy and light chains), linked so that the whole structure forms a 'Y' shape.

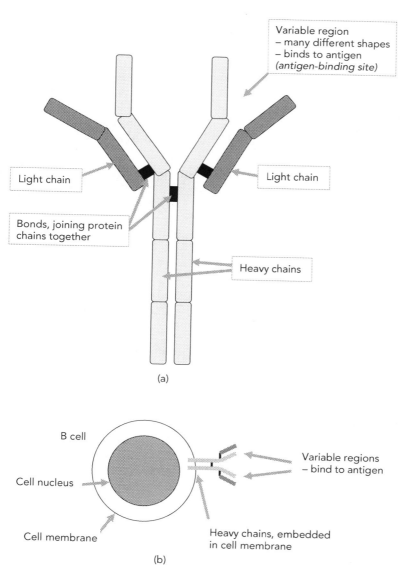

Variable region
– many different shapes
– binds to antigen
(antigen-binding site)

Light chain

Light chain

Bonds, joining protein
chains together

Heavy chains

(a)

B cell

Cell nucleus

Cell membrane

Variable regions
– bind to antigen

Heavy chains, embedded
in cell membrane

(b)

Box 5.4 (a) (*Continued*) Diagram of an antibody (immunoglobulin). (b) Diagrammatic representation of an immunoglobulin on the surface of a B cell, acting as an antigen receptor for the cell

There are five different groups of antibody (called *isotypes*) in mammals, which are classified according to the type of heavy chain they possess. Each of the groups performs slightly different roles in the body, ensuring the immune system responds appropriately to each type of 'foreign' material encountered by the body.

Most of the structure of different antibodies is similar; however, a region at the tip of the arms of the 'Y' shape varies and this variability of the tip structure means that millions of different antibodies exist.

This variable region recognises and binds very specifically to a distinct part of an antigen. The antigen-binding site is the cleft between the tip of a light chain and a heavy one. The highly specific binding means that antibodies identify and attach only to their target antigen and the many variants of antibody allow for an enormous range of different antibodies. Thus the immune system recognises a huge number of different antigens.

When an antibody recognises and attaches to an antigen it labels the antigen for attack by other parts of the immune system. Antibodies can also directly inhibit the harmful effects of an infectious agent by binding to it and blocking vital parts of the pathogen that it needs to cause an infection in the host.

Antibodies are either attached to B cells (*immunoglobulins*) or are secreted in soluble form into body fluids by plasma cells, which develop from stimulated B cells.

When antibodies (immunoglobulins, Igs) are fixed on the surface of B cells by their heavy chains (the bottom of the 'Y' shape), the variable antigen-binding sites stick out (bottom diagram) and are able to bind antigen. Thus, the Igs act as receptors which recognise specific foreign antigens. When a B cell comes into contact with an antigen which 'fits' its Ig receptors, it is prompted to start proliferating and its offspring are stimulated to produce more antibodies.

therefore blocking a part of the pathogen that it needs in order to cause an infection in the host.

Antibodies are either attached to B cells (in which case, strictly speaking, they are referred to as immunoglobulins) or are secreted in soluble form into body fluids by plasma cells, which develop from stimulated B cells. When antibodies (immunoglobulins) are fixed on the surface of B cells, their heavy chains (the bottom of the 'Y' shape) are embedded in the cell membrane so leaving the variable antigen-binding sites sticking out, and therefore able to bind antigen (see the bottom diagram of Box 5.4). Thus, the B cells in effect have receptors on their cell surfaces which recognise specific foreign antigens. When a B cell comes into contact with an antigen which 'fits' its receptors it is prompted (assisted by another type of lymphocyte called a T helper cell – more later) to start dividing. This means that one B cell makes many similar 'offspring' cells (called a *clone* of cells) that are capable of making more identical antibody to that produced by the original B cell. Thus the output of that particular antibody is greatly increased.

Plasma cells develop from antigen-stimulated B cells in the lymph nodes and spleen. When fully developed, the plasma cells migrate away from these areas and travel around the body. Plasma cells are antibody factories, able to secrete many thousands of antibody molecules each second! The antibody they produce is identical in antigen-specificity to the surface receptor (immunoglobulin) of the original 'parent' B cell (Box 5.5). Thus, all the new antibodies produced recognise the same antigen that triggered the B cells to proliferate in the first place.

After the initial stimulation by the antigen, the B cell response dies down but the antibody-producing cells have 'memory', and when the antigen is encountered on subsequent occasions, these specific B cells will respond more quickly and to a greater extent. So animals are said to have 'become immune' to a disease they have previously recovered from. This is also the basis of vaccination; when the vaccinated animal subsequently encounters the infectious organism against which it was vaccinated, it will mount a rapid and strong immune response and avoid development of disease.

Earlier we noted that different groups or classes (isotypes) of antibodies have slightly differing roles in the body. Some immunoglobulin classes are predominantly associated with certain areas of the body or are important in fighting certain types of pathogen. You may come across reference to the different immunoglobulin classes in your further reading; you may, for instance, hear about immunoglobulins G or A (or IgG or IgA as they are usually abbreviated). These letters denote the different classes of immunoglobulin and, for your information, the major roles of the classes are summarised in Box 5.6. Note that there are structural differences between the classes of immunoglobulin (not related to the variation in the antigen-receptor) and this means that some classes are bigger molecules than others, and this affects their roles.

Complement

Antibodies themselves cannot kill invading microorganisms; they simply label the organism so that another part of the immune system can destroy it. One important mechanism for this destruction of antibody-labelled microbes is the *complement* system. The complement system is a system of proteins which, when triggered, forms a chain or cascade, each protein being converted from an inactive to an active (enzyme) form; this active form then activates the next protein in the chain. It is a similar arrangement of the blood clotting cascade (see Chapter 7). One of the triggers for the complement protein cascade is the binding of antibody to antigen.

Box 5.5 The production of an antibody-secreting plasma cell from an antigen-stimulated B cell

When a B cell comes into contact with an antigen which 'fits' its surface receptors (specific immunoglobulin), it is prompted to start proliferating and its offspring are stimulated to produce more antibodies with the same antigen specificity.

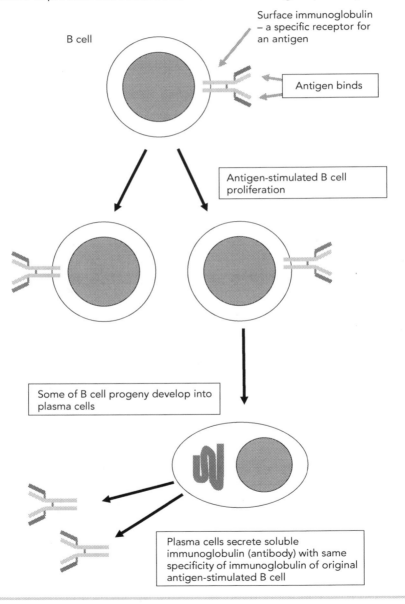

B cell

Surface immunoglobulin – a specific receptor for an antigen

Antigen binds

Antigen-stimulated B cell proliferation

Some of B cell progeny develop into plasma cells

Plasma cells secrete soluble immunoglobulin (antibody) with same specificity of immunoglobulin of original antigen-stimulated B cell

Box 5.5 (*Continued*) The production of an antibody-secreting plasma cell from an antigen-stimulated B cell

Plasma cells develop from antigen-stimulated B cells in the lymph nodes and spleen. When they are fully developed, the plasma cells leave these tissues and travel around the body.

Plasma cells are able to secrete vast numbers of antibody molecules. The antibody they produce is identical in antigen-specificity to the surface receptor (immunoglobulin) of the original 'parent' B cell. Thus all the new antibodies produced recognise the same antigen that triggered the parent B cell to proliferate.

The antibody response to an antigen has 'memory' which persists after the initial stimulation by the antigen dies down. When the antigen is encountered the next time, and on subsequent occasions, the specific B cells will respond more quickly and to a greater extent. These animals are said to have 'become immune' to a disease they have previously recovered from. This is also the basis of vaccination; when a vaccinated animal encounters the infectious organism against which it was vaccinated, it will mount a rapid and strong immune response, and the clinical signs of the disease will not develop.

The result of the cascade is that target cells carrying the antigenic molecule, perhaps because they are infected by microorganisms, are killed by damage to their cell membranes by the final stage of the complement system.

Another result of the complement system is that microbes may be clumped together and immobilised by the complement proteins making them vulnerable to attack by phagocytic cells.

Finally, complement is involved in inflammation by various direct and indirect (via mast cell stimulation) effects on blood vessel walls, and on white blood cell (neutrophil and macrophage) recruitment and activation (see Box 5.7) (see also Chapter 4 to remind yourself of the vascular and cellular events in acute inflammation).

Now let us turn our attention to the other lymphocyte family.

The T cell line

T cells originate in bone marrow but mature in the thymus (hence T cells!). The thymus is an organ in front of the heart in the chest (and sometimes the ventral neck) in very young animals. The thymus gradually shrinks, and almost disappears altogether, as the animal grows up. Mature T cells are found in the lymph nodes and spleen, but they also circulate throughout the body (see Box 5.8).

Remember how B cells carried immunoglobulins on their cell membranes and that these then acted as specific receptors for recognising

Box 5.6 The roles of different classes of immunoglobulins (antibodies)

	Found	Major roles or activities
IgG	In serum	Inflammation (very small molecule so can escape from leaky vessels – see Chapter 4), especially where microbes are involved.
IgM	In serum (soluble form) Also on surface of B cells	Very large molecule, so stays in bloodstream and is involved in defending against viruses and in a number of other aspects of the immune response. B cell antigen receptor.
IgA	On body surfaces (urinary, respiratory tracts, skin, mammary gland and intestine)	Passes through epithelial cells on body surfaces in secretions and fluids (also enters bloodstream). Helps to prevent antigens attaching to body surfaces.
IgE	On body surfaces	Usually acts with other cells and components of immune system to trigger acute inflammation. Involved in defence against parasitic worms. Involved in type I hypersensitivity (see later).
IgD	Only in some species Primarily on surface of B cells Serum (soluble form)	B cell antigen receptor.

In mammals there are five different groups of antibody, known as *isotypes*, classified according to the type of heavy chain they have. Each of the groups performs different roles in the body and helps the immune system to tailor its response to each type of antigen the body encounters. This table summarises the different types of antibody and indicate where they tend to be found and what sort of immune response they are associated with.

Note that IgM and IgD (in species which have it) act as B cell receptors.

There are structural differences between the classes of immunoglobulin which are not related to the variation in the antigen receptor. This means that some classes are bigger molecules than others, and this affects their roles.

antigen? T cells also have specific antigen receptors on their cell surfaces. T cell receptors are related to, but not the same as, B cell receptors. In other words, they are not actually immunoglobulins but they are similar in some ways and they make each T cell specific in their response to antigen.

The antigen is 'presented' to the T cells by other cells called antigen-presenting cells. Cells which can act as antigen-presenting cells include our old friends macrophages, also B cells, and another type of cell which we have only mentioned in passing so far – the *dendritic cells*.

Dendritic cells have long processes, a bit like cellular arms (see Box 5.8(b)); they can also live for a very long time.

So, the T cells are waiting in the lymphoid organs (lymph nodes and spleen) for the antigen-presenting cells to arrive with antigen that they 'found' in the nearby tissues. The antigen-presenting cells may take the microorganisms inside themselves by phagocytosis, but then they 'process' the antigen and carry it on their surfaces so that it can be recognised by cells of the immune system. The antigen-presenting cells carry the antigen to the lymphoid organs where they 'show it' to the T cell. If the T cell has the correct antigen receptor and 'recognises' the antigen as something foreign or harmful, it will respond by initiating an immune response.

The T cells which respond in this way are known as T helper cells because they 'help' the immune response in a number of ways. First, T helper cells encourage B cell proliferation and immunoglobulin secretion by secretion of chemical messengers which direct the B cells.

T helper cells also stimulate another type of T cell, called a *cytotoxic T cell*, whose role, once activated by the T helper cell, is to directly destroy any host cells harbouring the offending antigen. Note that the 'toxic' part of cytotoxic means 'damaging' rather than being a reference to a toxin or poison (and 'cyto-' indicates that the damage is aimed at cells).

Why should T cells want to damage cells? Well, if the stimulating antigen is a virus or a bacterium, then any cell infected with that organism will carry the antigen on its surface – a sort of label that says that the cell is infected.

Box 5.7 Diagram of the complement system

The complement system is a system of proteins which, when triggered (e.g. by the binding of antibody to antigen), form a chain or cascade, each protein being converted from an *inactive* to an *active* (enzyme) form. The active form then activates the next protein in the chain. The complement system is a similar arrangement to the blood clotting cascade (see Chapter 7).

The result of the complement cascade is (i) target cells carrying the antigenic molecule, perhaps because they are infected by microorganisms, are killed by damage to their cell membranes by the final stage of the complement system; (ii) microbes are clumped together and immobilised by the proteins, making them vulnerable to attack by phagocytic cells; (iii) complement is involved in acute inflammation by direct and indirect effects on blood vessel walls and on white blood cell recruitment and activation (see Chapter 4 to remind yourself of the protective role of acute inflammation).

Box 5.7 (*Continued*) Diagram of the complement system

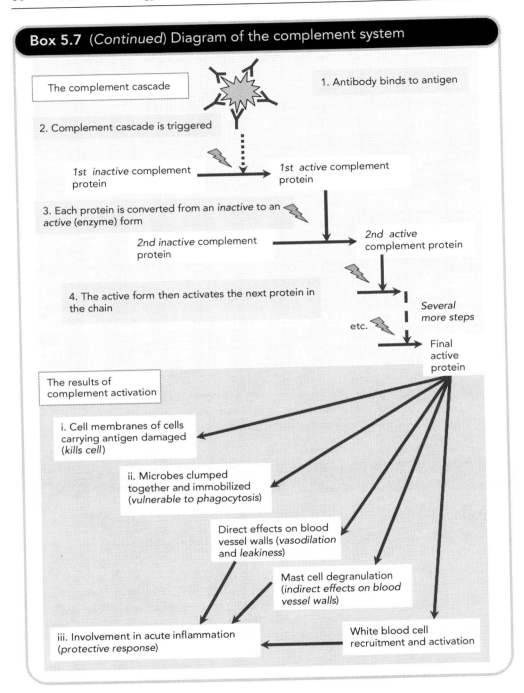

The complement cascade

1. Antibody binds to antigen

2. Complement cascade is triggered

1st *inactive* complement protein → 1st *active* complement protein

3. Each protein is converted from an *inactive* to an *active* (enzyme) form

2nd *inactive* complement protein → 2nd *active* complement protein

4. The active form then activates the next protein in the chain

etc.   Several more steps

Final active protein

The results of complement activation

i. Cell membranes of cells carrying antigen damaged (*kills cell*)

ii. Microbes clumped together and immobilized (*vulnerable to phagocytosis*)

Direct effects on blood vessel walls (*vasodilation* and *leakiness*)

Mast cell degranulation (*indirect effects on blood vessel walls*)

iii. Involvement in acute inflammation (*protective response*)

White blood cell recruitment and activation

As mentioned earlier, some tumour cells often carry abnormalities which are recognised by T cells and can act as antigen to stimulate the T cells, so in some cases the body will mount an immune response to tumours (see Chapter 8).

Stimulated cytotoxic T cells leave the lymphoid organs and set off to seek out antigen and kill the cells associated with it, such as cells infected with virus or bacteria, or tumour cells, by producing proteins which directly or indirectly cause the death of the infected cell.

We noted in our discussion on B cells that there is an element of 'memory' involved, so that the next time that particular antigen is encountered the B cell response will ensue more quickly and will be greater in intensity. The same aspect applies to T cell responses; to this end cells known as *memory T cells* persist after an immune response to a particular antigen has subsided.

The immune responses which involve activation and action of cells (macrophages, NK cells, antigen-specific cytotoxic T lymphocytes), and the release of various chemical messengers (called *cytokines*) are classified as *cell-mediated immunity* (CMI). CMI does not involve antibodies or complement. The part of the immune system which does involve antibodies is known as *humoral immunity*, from the Latin word 'humor' meaning *fluid*. Humoral immunity refers to the ability of body fluids,

Box 5.8 (a) The T cell family of lymphocytes

T cells originate in bone marrow, but mature in the thymus in young animals. Mature T cells are found in the lymph nodes and spleen, but they also circulate around the body.

T cells have specific antigen receptors on their cell surfaces (Box 5.8(b)), similar to, but not the same as, B cell receptors (see Box 5.4).

Antigen-presenting cells (macrophages, dendritic cells or B cells) 'find' antigen in the nearby tissues and return with it to the lymphoid organs (lymph nodes and spleen). Here they 'present' the antigen to the T cells. If the T cell has the appropriate antigen receptor and 'recognises' the antigen it responds by initiating an immune response. The T cells which respond in this way are known as T helper cells and they secrete chemical messengers (cytokines) which stimulate B cell proliferation and immunoglobulin secretion. T helper cells also prompt cytotoxic T cells into action; the role of cytotoxic T cells is to destroy other cells harbouring the offending antigen.

Stimulated cytotoxic T cells leave the lymphoid organs and set off to seek out and destroy the antigen and the cells associated with it.

Cytotoxic T cells kill these other cells by inserting lethal proteins through the outer membrane of the target cell.

As with B cells and the humoral response, there is 'memory' involved in the T cell response by the generation of memory T cells, which will respond more quickly and with greater intensity the next time that the particular antigen is encountered.

Box 5.8 (a) (*Continued*) The T cell family of lymphocytes

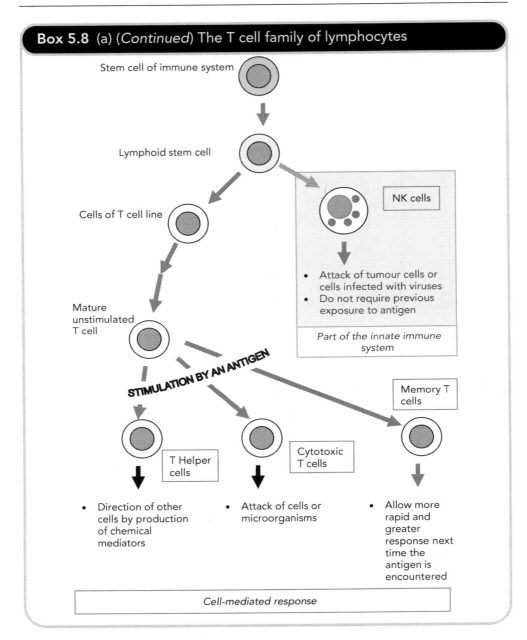

Stem cell of immune system

Lymphoid stem cell

Cells of T cell line

Mature
unstimulated
T cell

NK cells

- Attack of tumour cells or
  cells infected with viruses
- Do not require previous
  exposure to antigen

*Part of the innate immune
system*

STIMULATION BY AN ANTIGEN

Memory T
cells

T Helper
cells

Cytotoxic
T cells

- Direction of other
  cells by production
  of chemical
  mediators

- Attack of cells or
  microorganisms

- Allow more
  rapid and
  greater
  response next
  time the
  antigen is
  encountered

Cell-mediated response

which do not necessarily contain cells, to mount an immune response
(which they do because of the presence of antibodies).

Note that not just T helper cells, but many cells of the immune system the chemical messangers *cytokines* and that these direct and en-
hance other aspects of the immune response, and direct both humoral

Box 5.8 (b) (Continued) The actions of stimulated T cells

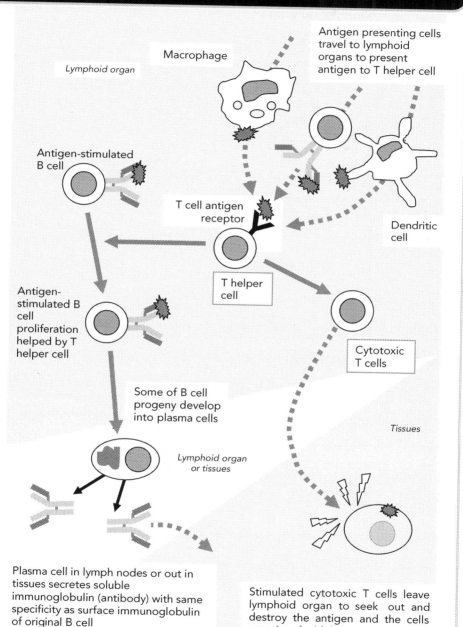

Plasma cell in lymph nodes or out in tissues secretes soluble immunoglobulin (antibody) with same specificity as surface immunoglobulin of original B cell

Stimulated cytotoxic T cells leave lymphoid organ to seek out and destroy the antigen and the cells associated with it

and cellular responses. Many cytokines bridge the gap between immunity and inflammation as they direct aspects of both processes.

Natural killer cells

In our discussion of the innate immune system earlier in the chapter, we heard about a type of lymphocyte with the curious name of *natural killer cell*! These probably develop from the same cell line as the T cell family of lymphocytes (see Box 5.8) but they are different in their actions. NK cells are large lymphocytes with abundant granules in their cytoplasm, hence their alternative (but less exciting) name of *large granular lymphocytes*. NK cells act as part of the *innate immune system* since they have the ability to rapidly destroy certain abnormal cells such as tumour cells and cells infected with viruses. They do not require 'priming' by previous encounters with the abnormal cells, as do their more sophisticated cousins the T cells or their distant relatives the B cells.

That concludes our very simplified discussion of the normal immune system. Box 5.9 contains a diagrammatic summary and it might be helpful to look again at Boxes 5.1–5.8 as well before you read on. There may be terms in those boxes that now become clearer.

Diseases of the immune system

Disorders of reduced immune function

Immunodeficiencies

We now turn our attention to what can go wrong with the immune responses, and we start with diseases associated with reduced function of the immune system. As you might imagine, disorders causing reduced immunity cause increased vulnerability to disease in the affected animal. These disorders are divided into *primary disorders* – those associated with inherited defects in the immune system – and *secondary disorders* – those resulting from another disease, disorder or condition which secondarily cause a decrease in immune function.

Primary immunodeficiency

Primary immunodeficiencies are uncommon congenital disorders in animals, but may be suspected when there are persistent or repeated bouts of infectious disease in young animals especially where unusual *pathogens* are involved. Affected animals may remain healthy whilst they are still protected by antibodies passed to them by their mothers (that is whilst they were developing in the uterus or after birth via mother's milk). When their mother's protection stops they become vulnerable to disease.

Box 5.9 Summary of the immune responses

A. Foreign substance carrying antigenic molecule negotiates physical barriers to enter body. Some will not actually enter the body but remain on the surface (perhaps stuck in mucus) and will attract antibodies and white cells in secretions.

B. Components of the innate immune system may be able to disable and destroy substance. Natural killer cells can rapidly, but non-specifically, respond to and destroy cells infected with viruses, or certain tumour cells.

C. Antigen-presenting cells, macrophages, dendritic cells and B cells ingest foreign material and 'process' the antigen molecule, displaying it on their cell surfaces. They then carry it back to a lymphoid tissue, such as a local lymph node. B cells which act as antigen-presenting cells have immunoglobulin on their surfaces which is specific for the antigen, recognising only that antigen molecule.

D. In the lymphoid tissue the antigen-presenting cells 'show' the antigen molecule to an appropriate T helper cell, that is, a T helper cell with a surface receptor which 'fits' the antigen.

E. The T helper cell stimulates antigen-specific B cells to proliferate. Antigen-specific B cells have immunoglobulin on their surface which 'fits' the antigen too.

F. Some of the daughter cells of the stimulated B cell become plasma cells. In the lymph nodes and out in the tissues, the plasma cells start to secrete antibodies of the same specificity as the surface immunoglobulin receptor of the original stimulated B cell.

G. Secreted antibodies bind to antigen molecules, labelling them for other parts of the immune system.

H. Binding of antigen and antibody triggers the cascade of complement proteins.

I. The final product of complement cascade is able to clump and immobilise microbes, stimulate inflammation (a protective response) and kill cells carrying antigen.

J. The T helper cell in the lymph node also stimulates cytotoxic T cells.

K. Cytotoxic T cells travel out of the lymph node and seek out and kill cells carrying the antigen molecule.

Both the B cell and T cell arms of the immune response have memory so that the next time this particular antigen is encountered, they can respond more quickly and to a greater extent.

Box 5.9 (Continued) Summary of the immune responses

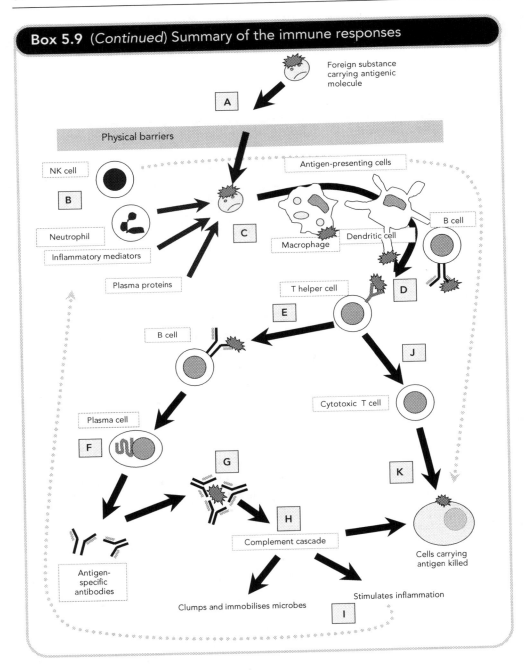

Foreign substance carrying antigenic molecule

A

Physical barriers

NK cell

B

Neutrophil

Inflammatory mediators

Plasma proteins

C

Antigen-presenting cells

Macrophage

Dendritic cell

B cell

D

T helper cell

E

B cell

J

Cytotoxic T cell

Plasma cell

F

G

H

K

Complement cascade

Cells carrying antigen killed

Antigen-specific antibodies

Clumps and immobilises microbes

Stimulates inflammation

I

Such animals also fail to respond to vaccinations which require an immune response to work against common diseases, and treatment for the infections may be unsuccessful or only partially successful. These animals will often have abnormal haematology (unusually low or high white cell counts) or blood biochemistry (abnormal globulin levels).

Examples of mechanisms of primary immunodeficiencies include abnormalities in immunoglobulins, cells (neutrophils, macrophages or lymphocytes) or in complement proteins. Well-known examples of primary immunodeficiency diseases are the group of diseases known as severe combined immunodeficiencies (or SCID) in certain breeds of dogs and horses, and in mice, in which several types of lymphocytes are affected.

Confirmation of a primary immunodeficiency requires specialist tests, which are not readily available in general veterinary practice and usually require referral to an immunologist.

Treatment of primary immunodeficiencies is difficult because of the inherent vulnerability to disease of an animal with such a disorder. Symptomatic treatment and anti-microbial treatment may provide temporary relief but the longer-term prognosis is very poor.

Secondary immunodeficiency

Secondary immunodeficiencies are disorders which occur secondarily to some other disease, disorder or physiological condition.

Some important conditions associated with secondary immunodeficiency are:

- *Physiological states*: Age, breed, gender, pregnancy, season of the year, stress and trauma, diet and hormones are all known or believed to affect immune function in animals. Suppression of the immune system occurs during pregnancy; indeed, this mechanism aims to stop the mother rejecting the developing embryo. A side effect of this, however, is the likelihood that, for instance, *Demodex* skin mites in bitches will multiply during pregnancy and lactation and then be transmitted to the puppies.
- *Chronic diseases*: Chronic diseases appear to interfere with function of cells, such as lymphocytes or neutrophils. The sorts of diseases implicated in immune suppression include various infections, especially long-term skin infections, and viruses. Some viruses (such as canine distemper and feline infectious peritonitis (FIP)) cause immunosuppression because they tend to proliferate in, and ultimately destroy, lots of cells involved in the immune responses (such as lymphocytes).

Two other important viruses that suppress the immune system are feline immunodeficiency virus (FIV) and feline leukaemia virus

(FeLV). FIV has several effects on infected cats (such as tumour formation and neurological disease) but, importantly for the purposes of this discussion, it causes immunosuppression in these cats. It has its immunosuppressive action by targeting T lymphocytes, similar to the human (and primate) condition of HIV AIDS. Affected cats then become susceptible to, and may die from, a number of other infectious agents which normally would not cause serious disease in animals with fully-functioning immune systems.

FeLV also causes loss of normal immune function. FeLV has detrimental effects on bone marrow (the source of many cells involved in immune and inflammatory responses) and, as with FIV, cats (and especially kittens) succumb to other infections, rather than to the leukaemia it also causes and which gives the virus its name. Bone marrow depletion causes anaemia as well and this may be detected clinically.

- *Drugs and vaccines*: Certain administered drugs are implicated in immunodeficiency states. Examples of this are the glucocorticoids (corticosteroids) which have anti-inflammatory effects but also diminish the immune response whilst the animal is on treatment due to effects on neutrophils, macrophages and lymphocytes. Rarely, certain vaccines cause a transient decrease in lymphocyte numbers in the blood (*lymphopenia*) which potentially could make an animal more vulnerable to other infections for a short while. This is partly the reason we try to make sure that we only vaccinate animals that are clinically healthy, and advise that puppies and kittens are kept away from possible sources of infection (i.e. other animals) for a period after vaccination.
- *Neoplasia*: Occasionally, animals have abnormalities of immunoglobulin formation (and function). This can occur with certain tumours of plasma cells. Abnormal (and non-functional) immunoglobulins accumulate in the blood and urine and can be detected in the laboratory.
- *Failure of passive immunity*: Young animals gain immunity from their mothers by transfer of the mother's antibodies during their time in the womb, or by the consumption of colostrum within 12–48 hours after birth (a process known as *passive immune* protection). Passive immunity is especially important for protection of the newborn animal from potential pathogens in their environment before they are able to mount an effective immune response for themselves (see Box 5.10).

Animals that do not consume sufficient colostrum, perhaps because they are too weak to stand, or their mothers are too poorly to allow

Box 5.10 Passive immune protection of young animals

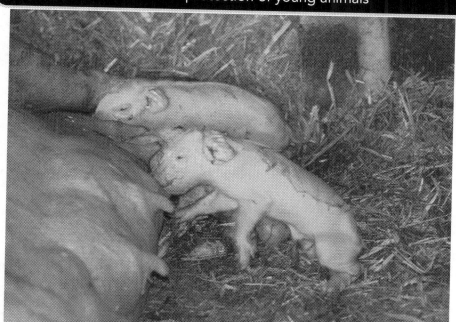

Newborn piglets, still coated with foetal fluids and membranes, demonstrate the strong instinct to find their mother's teats as soon as possible after birth.

Young animals gain immunity from their mothers by transfer of the mother's antibodies during pregnancy, or by consuming the rich first-milk – colostrum – soon after birth (a process known as passive immune protection). Passive immunity is especially important for protecting the young animal from environmental infections before they are able to mount an effective immune response themselves. Young animals that drink insufficient colostrum, perhaps because they are too weak to stand, or their mothers are too poorly to let them suck, are vulnerable to early infections, especially if the environment is contaminated.

Photograph courtesy of Joe Brownlie. Sow and piglets photographed by kind permission of Helen Wakeham.

suckling, may be vulnerable to infections early in life, especially if the environment is dirty and contaminated.

The previous discussion involves disorders due to insufficient function of the immune system. Diseases also occur if the immune system works too much or works inappropriately and these two mechanisms form the basis of the disorders discussed in the next two sections – *hypersensitivities* and *autoimmunity*.

Disorders of increased or inappropriate immunity

Hypersensitivities

As the name of these conditions suggests, hypersensitivities (or hypersensitivity reactions) are excessive reactions mediated by the immune system to stimuli which would not be harmful in a normal animal. If you are a hay fever sufferer you will recognise this syndrome. Something like pollen grains will make you have the miserable signs of itchy, runny eyes and persistent sneezing at certain times of the year, whereas others in your family or circle of friends will be unaffected. This type of hypersensitivity is classed as an *allergy* but other types are also recognised and each has a slightly different mechanism. The four types of hypersensitivity are classed as types one, two, three and four and are conventionally written with a Roman numeral (I, II, III and IV). In reality, clinical syndromes involving hypersensitivity reactions will often involve more than one of the types I–IV.

Each type of hypersensitivity is described below and Box 5.11 is a brief summary of each type and its mechanism; you may find it helpful to refer back to the discussion of the normal immune system to understand these mechanisms of hypersensitivity.

Type I hypersensitivity

Type I hypersensitivity is also known as *immediate hypersensitivity* and it is the basis of acute *allergic responses*. In this hypersensitivity response, *antigens* (or *allergens*) to which the animal is sensitised cause specific *antibodies* (*immunoglobulins*) to stimulate *mast cells* to degranulate. Degranulation means that the stimulated mast cells release the contents of their intracytoplasmic granules.

Reminder

Contents of mast cell granules include histamine, a potent biological chemical, which has a number of actions, including the ability to stimulate *endothelial* cell contraction. This action opens up gaps between the endothelial cells in the capillary walls, allowing escape of protein-rich *exudate* into surrounding tissues. Histamine also causes vasodilation (see Chapter 4).

After reminding yourself of the properties of mast cells in the text box above (and from our discussion of mast cells from Chapter 4) you will predict that the effects of mast cell degranulation are dilation of nearby blood vessels and seepage of oedema fluid and proteins (*exudate*) and, later, influx of inflammatory cells to the area. There may be

Box 5.11 The four categories of hypersensitivity disease

Hypersensitivities (or hypersensitivity reactions) are excessive or inappropriate reactions mediated by the immune system in response to stimuli that would be relatively unimportant in a normal animal. Hypersensitivities are classified as four types and each type is conventionally designated a Roman numeral (I, II, III and IV). In reality, clinical syndromes involving hypersensitivity reactions will often involve more than one of the types I–IV occurring together.

Each type is described in the text whilst this box is a brief summary of each type and its mechanism.

Type	Mechanism	Example of disease
I	Immunoglobulins stimulate marked mast cell degranulation	Anaphylactic shock Food allergies (skin or GIT disease) Reaction to insect bite or sting
II	Antibodies inappropriately label cells of the body as 'foreign' or 'harmful'. Target cells then killed by other parts of the immune system	Blood transfusion reactions
III	Damage caused to tissue by accumulation of antigen–antibody–complement protein complexes	Widespread pyogranulomatous inflammation centred on blood vessels in feline infectious peritonitis
IV	T helper lymphocytes direct immune response to cells	Allergic contact dermatitis

additional effects, depending on where the mast cell response occurs, for instance, in the respiratory tract the smooth muscle surrounding the airways also constricts impairing airflow in the airways (as in asthma). In the skin, nerve endings are stimulated and so there is extreme itchiness (*pruritus*).

The effects of mast cell degranulation in type I hypersensitivity can sometimes be more widespread than a particular area, leading to generalised *anaphylaxis*. Anaphylaxis is a very sudden, severe, life-threatening, generalised allergic or type I hypersensitivity reaction, to a stimulus to which the host is especially sensitive. Anaphylaxis causes shock – a severe acute fall in blood pressure (see Chapter 7).

Eosinophils tend to be present in type I hypersensitivity reactions as they are attracted to degranulating mast cells. Once attracted to the area, eosinophils may then release the contents of their own intracytoplasmic granules and cause tissue damage and secondary inflammation. The feline *eosinophilic granuloma complex mentioned* in Chapter 4 is also thought to be a form of type I hypersensitivity.

Type II hypersensitivity

Also known as *cytotoxic* hypersensitivity, type II hypersensitivity is an immune response in which elements of the immune system are directed to kill cells of the body. This occurs because the target cells have been inappropriately labelled with antibodies as 'foreign' or 'harmful'. (Remember that 'cytotoxic' means something that is very damaging to cells but does not imply a toxin or poison is involved. Remember also that antibodies coat substances – including cells – to label them for destruction by other parts of the immune system.)

A reasonably common example of a type II hypersensitivity response of clinical significance is immune-mediated destruction of red cells causing anaemia, as happens in blood transfusion reactions.

Type III hypersensitivity

In this type of hypersensitivity response, tissue damage results from the accumulation of *antigen*, *antibody* and *complement proteins* – forming protein clumps called *antibody* or *immune complexes*. Clumps of *antigen*, *antibody* and proteins of the *complement* cascade actually form in most immune responses but they are usually ultimately destroyed by *phagocytic* cells. When there has been excessive immune stimulation, the complexes can build up and resist degradation. The immune complexes may remain at their site of formation or they may circulate in the blood stream and lodge in other tissues. Wherever they form the presence of these immune complexes stimulates local *inflammation* which then causes damage to the surrounding tissues.

Excessive formation of immune complexes can occur in certain infectious diseases such as FIP in which inflammation, mostly *pyogranulomatous* (*pyo*granulomatous means granulomas with neutrophils as well as macrophages in the centre – see Chapter 4) is centred on small blood vessels (vasculitis) in many organs, causing widespread vascular damage.

Type IV hypersensitivity

Also known as *delayed-type hypersensitivity*, this hypersensitivity is essentially an inflammatory response, involving cells of the immune system, which can take several hours (24–72 hours) to develop after the sensitised animal is exposed to the stimulus to which it is sensitive. The immune cells involved in triggering delayed-type hypersensitivity are T helper cells; there is also activation of macrophages and B lymphocytes. More macrophages, lymphocytes and also neutrophils are subsequently recruited via chemical messengers (cytokines) secreted by the initially stimulated immune cells and hence the delay in manifestation of the response.

Allergic contact dermatitis is an example of such a response, and the cause of the response may be identified by carrying out a patch test on the skin of the animal. A patch test involves applying small samples of suspect allergens to an area of skin and seeing whether there is a local response.

Autoimmune disorders

Autoimmune disorders occur when the immune system mounts an immune response against the body's own tissues because normal proteins on the surface of cells are regarded as 'foreign'. There are various reasons why this attack of the body's own cells may occur and mechanisms, including failure of regulatory control of the immune system or new exposure of self-antigens that are normally in protected sites, 'hidden' away from the immune system (such as in the eye), may be involved. Certain viruses may trigger autoimmunity by mimicking normal proteins, or by other means of which we are not quite sure!

There are a number of autoimmune disorders in veterinary species, including the pemphigus complex of skin diseases. In these diseases, which occur in dogs, cats, goats and horses, the immune attack is directed at proteins in the epidermis, or epithelial surface of the skin. The epidermal layer is killed off and therefore these diseases are characterised by blistering, *erosion* and *ulceration*, of the skin and mucocutaneous junctions.

Another disease in this category is autoimmune haemolytic anaemia (AIHA) which is recorded in a number of species but mostly occurs in dogs. Affected animals present with clinical signs associated with severe anaemia such as pallor, breathlessness and weakness. Their spleens may be enlarged and they have rapid heartbeats (tachycardia). The cause of AIHA is not entirely understood but may relate to alterations in the surface of red blood cells by other factors such as drugs or viruses. Some cases seem to be associated with stresses of various kinds, such as other diseases or pregnancy, for instance.

Masticatory myopathy is an autoimmune disorder in which the immune response is directed against the muscle fibres of the masticatory (chewing) muscles of the head of large dogs. These animals have difficulty opening and closing their jaws and the sides of their heads may be painful and either swollen or shrunken (muscle *atrophy* – see Chapter 8). They may have associated abnormalities in their eyes such as inflammation (conjunctivitis) or even protrusion of the eyeballs from the eye sockets.

Treatment of autoimmune diseases (in those conditions able to be treated) relies on controlling the inappropriate immune response by dampening down the immune system. This can have the unwanted effect, however, of leaving the animal vulnerable to other diseases, especially infections.

Summary of key points in Chapter 5

- The body's defences against harmful invaders are composed of the innate and the adaptive immune systems; epithelial surfaces and associated protective devices also provide physical barrier defence for the body.
- The adaptive immune system is sub-divided into cellular (lymphocyte and macrophage) responses and humoral (antibody) responses.
- There are links between the immune system and the inflammatory responses also wound healing, since some cells are common to each response, also important chemical messengers (mediators) called cytokines are involved in all processes.
- The immune responses are protective but some disorders or diseases result from abnormal immune responses. Immunodeficiencies are due to decreased immune function. This may be primary (an inherited genetic disorder) or secondary to another disease or disorder (chronic disease, physiological factors, drugs or neoplasia).
- Hypersensitivities occur when the immune response overreacts or reacts inappropriately to a stimulus. There are four types of hypersensitivity with slightly differing mechanisms.
- Autoimmune diseases occur when the immune system directs its attack against a normal ('self') molecule and an immune response aimed at destroying the molecule ensues.

Test yourself questions on Chapter 5

1. List all the defences of animals against invading infectious organisms.

2. From which two words is the term 'antigen' derived?

3. Answer the following true/false questions relating to the immune system:

    i. Lymphocytes are small round cells with sparse cytoplasm and single round nuclei.
    ii. Lymphocytes are only found in organs of the lymphoid system.
    iii. Lymphocytic cells belong to the B cell line or the T cell line.
    iv. A major role of plasma cells is to phagocytose bacteria.
    v. T cell receptors and immunoglobulins on B cells make the cells specific in their response to antigen.
    vi. Antibodies are formed from paired chains of proteins in a 'Y' shape and it is the bonds joining the chains which make them specific to a particular antigen.
    vii. When a vaccinated animal encounters the infectious organism against which it was vaccinated, it will mount a rapid and strong immune response because the specific antibody-producing B cells have 'memory'.
    viii. Antibodies are able to kill invading microorganisms.
    ix. Cells called antigen-presenting cells are able to alert T cells called T helper cells to the presence of potentially harmful infectious organisms.
    x. Unlike B cells, T cell responses do not have 'memory' of previous encounters with particular antigens.

4. Some important conditions are associated with immunodeficiency; complete the following sentences:

    • Primary immunodeficiencies are suspected in cases of
    ....
    ....
    in young animals.
    • Physiological states such as
    ....
    ....
    are often associated with immunodeficiency.
    • Certain chronic diseases are associated with immunodeficiency, and this may be because they
    ....
    ....

Test yourself questions on Chapter 5 (*Continued*)

- With respect to young animals, passive immunity includes

  ....

  ....

  ....

  ....

- Failure of passive immunity in young animals can occur because

  ....

  ....

  ....

5. a. Give a brief definition of 'hypersensitivity'.
    b. Choose one type of hypersensitivity (type I, II, III or IV) and write brief notes on its characteristic features.

6. a. Give a brief definition of 'autoimmunity'.
    b. Briefly, what is the treatment or control of autoimmune diseases based upon, and what general side effect is possible?

Chapter 6
Tissue Repair

Definition of tissue repair or healing

Regenerative capacity of cells

Tissue repair – general and specific examples

Healing in various tissues

Liver
Kidney and lungs
Heart
Nervous system

Healing regulation and control

What can impair, prevent or alter healing?

Proud flesh

Definition of tissue repair or healing

Following damage, all tissues (except teeth) are able to heal to a certain extent. Tissue repair or healing is defined as the process by which cells lost by non-reversible cell damage (see necrosis, Chapter 3) are replaced by living tissue. This new living tissue is not necessarily the same as the tissue it is replacing. The extent to which the new tissue is the same as the tissue that was previously there depends on:

- the *regenerative capacity* of the cells in tissue
- the *extent* of the defect to be filled (that is the amount of necrotic tissue requiring replacement)

Two processes are involved in tissue healing:

1. *Regeneration*: Replacement by cells of the same type. The necrotic cells themselves are dead so they cannot regenerate. Instead, it is surrounding living cells which regenerate (if they are able to – see discussion of different cell types below) and fill in the gap left by the dead cells.
2. *Organisation*: Replacement by fibrovascular connective tissue (scar tissue). This occurs when cells are not able to regenerate themselves or where there has been a large area of necrosis, so living regenerative cells are further away from the centre of the area of damage or cannot fill the gap quickly enough.

Box 6.1 is a flow diagram to summarise tissue repair and we shall discuss the processes involved in this chapter.

Box 6.1 Flow diagram to simplify healing and repair

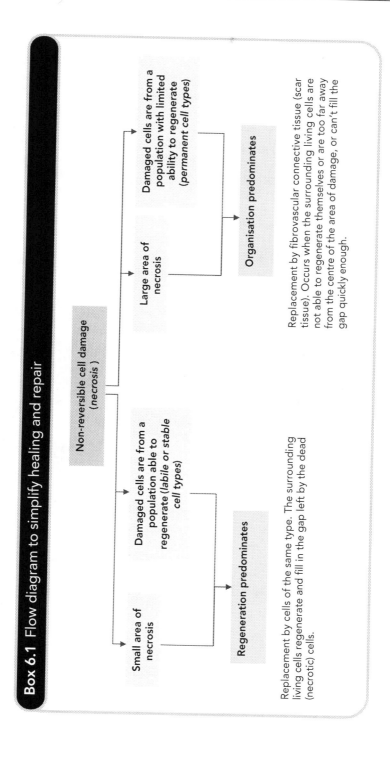

Non-reversible cell damage (necrosis)

Small area of necrosis → Damaged cells are from a population able to regenerate (labile or stable cell types) → **Regeneration predominates**

Replacement by cells of the same type. The surrounding living cells regenerate and fill in the gap left by the dead (necrotic) cells.

Large area of necrosis → Damaged cells are from a population with limited ability to regenerate (permanent cell types) → **Organisation predominates**

Replacement by fibrovascular connective tissue (scar tissue). Occurs when the surrounding living cells are not able to regenerate themselves or are too far away from the centre of the area of damage, or can't fill the gap quickly enough.

Regenerative capacity of cells

Cells are divided into *labile*, *stable* and *permanent* cell populations according to their ability to replace themselves (see Box 6.2).

In any one organ both of the processes of regeneration or organisation may occur due to the different cell types which make up each organ, e.g. liver is composed not just of liver cells, but also connective tissue cells and blood vessel endothelial cells; muscles contain not just muscle fibres, but also connective tissue, blood vessels, nerves and so on. One of the processes will tend to predominate, however, and which of the processes is most important in repair of a damaged organ depends on the ability of the main cells of the organ to replace themselves.

Regeneration

For damaged tissue to heal by regeneration, the cells that make it up must be able to divide by the process of *mitosis*. Cells vary in this ability and can be broadly categorised as labile, stable or permanent (see Box 6.2 for definitions and examples of the different cell

---

Box 6.2 Cell populations according to their ability to replace themselves

Labile cells:	Cells continue to multiply by mitosis throughout life and replace those lost due to normal turnover
Examples of labile cells:	Epidermal cells of the skin surface and intestinal epithelial cells, lymphoid cells of the immune system and haematopoietic (blood-producing) cells of bone marrow
Stable cells:	Have long life spans, do not normally turnover quickly but following tissue injury they rapidly divide to replace damaged cells
Examples of stable cells:	Epithelial cells in liver, kidney and lung
Permanent cells:	Have no or very limited capacity to regenerate new cells
Examples of permanent cells:	Neurons in brain and spinal cord and cardiac muscle cells
Note that there are also	
Stem cells:	Stem cells are present in labile and stable populations. After division, stem cells can differentiate according to the body's or tissue's requirements

populations). There are also cells known as stem cells, which can divide and differentiate along many different paths to form different mature cell types.

Organisation

In situations where cells are not able to regenerate themselves, because they are not labile or stable cell populations, or where the damage is just too great for them to do so, the area will repair by the process of organisation.

Organisation is divided into three phases: the *demolition* or *inflammatory* phase, the *granulation* phase and the *maturation* phase. These phases are discussed below. It should be borne in mind that the phases of organisation in a healing wound may overlap.

Phases of organisation (see Box 6.3)

- *Demolition or inflammatory* phase: In the demolition or inflammatory phase, 'cleaning-up' of the wound or damaged tissue occurs. This is performed mainly by neutrophils and macrophages, though lymphocytes, plasma cells and eosinophils may be involved under some circumstances. (See Chapter 4 for properties of neutrophils and other cells involved in inflammation.)
- *Granulation* phase: In the granulation phase immature connective tissue (*granulation tissue*) is formed to start to fill in the wound. Note that granulation tissue is not the same thing as granuloma formation (see chronic granulomatous inflammation in Chapter 4).
- *Maturation* phase: In the maturation phase the immature fibrous tissue formed in the phase of granulation matures by a process called fibrosis. The result of this phase is formation of a fibrous scar.

To appreciate the difference between the tissue formed in the last two phases of organisation, granulation tissue and fibrous tissue, see Box 6.4.

As you see from Box 6.4, the amount of granulation tissue, fibrosis and, therefore, scar formation depends on the extent of damage and therefore the size of the wound to be filled. In the next section, we discuss how different sorts of wounds are healed, using skin wounds as an example. We will then briefly discuss healing in some other major tissues in the body. Before we leave this section, however, Box 6.5 summarises what we have discussed so far.

Box 6.3 Diagrammatic representation of the phases of wound organisation

A skin wound is used as an example.

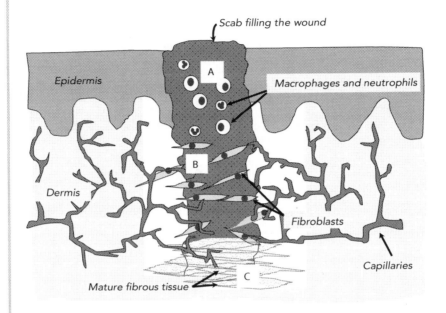

For simplicity, all phases are shown in one diagram – note that, in most wounds, there will be a gradual progression from one phase to the next as time goes on.

A. *Demolition* or *inflammatory* phase. This is the phase of 'cleaning-up' of the wound or damaged tissue, mainly by neutrophils and macrophages.

B. *Granulation* phase. In the granulation phase, immature connective tissue (*granulation tissue* formation) is formed to start to fill in the wound. Granulation tissue consists of immature fibre-producing cells (fibroblasts) and capillaries which grow into the area from adjacent tissue.

C. *Maturation* phase. This is the maturation of the immature fibrous tissue formed in the granulation phase by a process called fibrosis. The result of this phase is formation of a fibrous scar.

Box 6.4 The differences between granulation tissue and fibrous tissue

Granulation tissue

- Immature connective tissue
- Forms rapidly as a scaffold for stronger repair
- Amount depends on size of defect

Fibrous tissue

- Mature connective tissue
- Collagen (protein fibre)-rich
- Strong component of repair
- When fully mature fibrosis contracts (scar)
- Amount depends on size of defect

Tissue repair – general and specific examples

1. Healing where there has been *epithelial damage only* (Box 6.6): Using skin as our example, consider a minor and superficial skin wound where there has been damage only to the outermost layer (the epidermis). When the epidermis is damaged, there will be exudation of serum (see again acute inflammation, Chapter 4). This ooze will dry and harden to form a scab. Skin scab is dried serum protein (fibrin), sometimes with some dead and dying white cells,

Box 6.5 Summary of the introduction to tissue repair and wound healing

- Tissue healing or repair = the process by which necrotic cells are replaced by living tissue
- Most tissues are able to repair, but the new cells may not be the same as the cells they are replacing
- Regeneration = replacement by cells of the same type
- Organisation = replacement by fibrovascular connective tissue (scar tissue)
- The extent to which each of these processes occurs depends on:
  - How well the cells in the tissue are able to regenerate (*regenerative capacity*)
  - How big is the area of necrosis
- Cells are categorised as labile, stable and permanent according to their ability to divide (by mitosis, i.e. their regenerative capacity). There are also stem cells
- In many organs, both processes (regeneration and organisation) may occur due to different cell types which make up the tissue (e.g. epithelial cells and connective tissue cells)

such as neutrophils, stuck in the scab especially where there has been bacterial contamination of the wound. This scab serves to protect the next stage in the healing process. Underneath the dried scab there is proliferation of the epithelium (in our skin example, the proliferating epithelium will be epidermis – the top covering layer of skin) from around the edge of the wound. The epithelial cells proliferate readily by mitosis since they are labile cells (see earlier, this chapter).

The proliferating cells gradually move across to form a continuous layer beneath scab. Eventually, the scab falls away revealing the newly regenerated and healed epidermis beneath. In this case there is minimal granulation tissue and fibrosis (scar formation).

We have used skin in our example but note that the essentials of healing described are the same in other tissues that have an epithelial (covering) surface.

2. Healing of deeper or more severe wounds where *more than epithelium is affected*: Two types of healing are recognised in this situation, depending on the extent of the wound to be filled.
    a. Healing by *first intention* or *primary union* (see Box 6.7(a)): A good example of the sort of wound that would heal by first intention (or primary union) would be a clean, incised (surgical) wound. The wound will be deeper than just the epidermis but the edges of the wound will be neat and closely apposed (especially if sutured) and there should be no or very few bacteria present to contaminate the wound.

    The surface epidermis will regenerate as described above. Whilst underneath the epidermal layer a soft jelly-like protein plug of the serum protein, fibrin, will form. This will be replaced by a slender seam of granulation tissue in 5–7 days via organisation and by mature fibrosis (scar) in 2–3 weeks. Note these timings. This is why we tend to leave stitches in place for at least 10 days after most surgical procedures and why we suggest continued lead walking for dogs and restrict them from jumping up into cars or onto furniture for sometime afterwards.
    b. *Second intention/secondary union* or healing of a wound where there is a tissue defect (see Box 6.7(b)): Edges of wound are widely separated, tissue has been lost and the defect contains exudate and necrotic debris (and possibly bacterial contamination if the wound is not surgical). In this case the defect must again fill in by granulation, maturing to fibrosis, but more of it must form to fill the gap. As before, the fibrous tissue matures but this may take several weeks, and when it contracts

Box 6.6 Healing where there is epithelial damage only

Simplified diagrams of healing in a superficial and uncomplicated skin wound

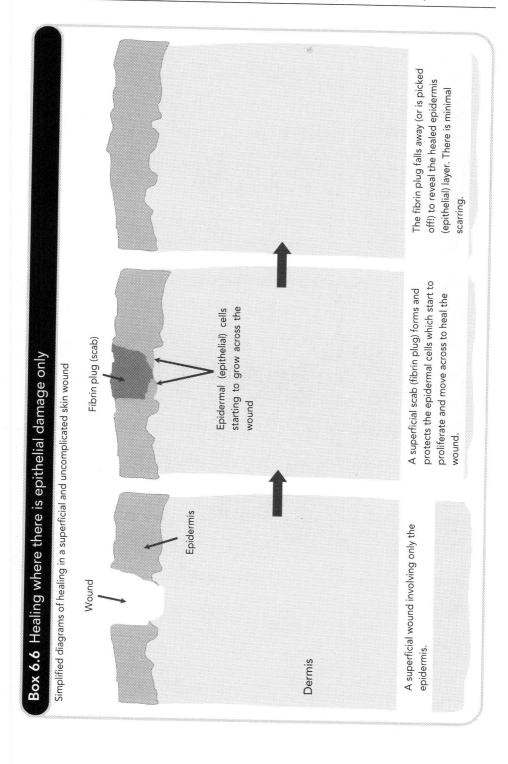

Wound

Fibrin plug (scab)

Epidermis

Dermis

Epidermal (epithelial) cells starting to grow across the wound

A superficial wound involving only the epidermis.

A superficial scab (fibrin plug) forms and protects the epidermal cells which start to proliferate and move across to heal the wound.

The fibrin plug falls away (or is picked off!) to reveal the healed epidermis (epithelial) layer. There is minimal scarring.

Box 6.7 (a) Healing by first intention

Simplified diagrams of first intention healing in a surgical skin wound

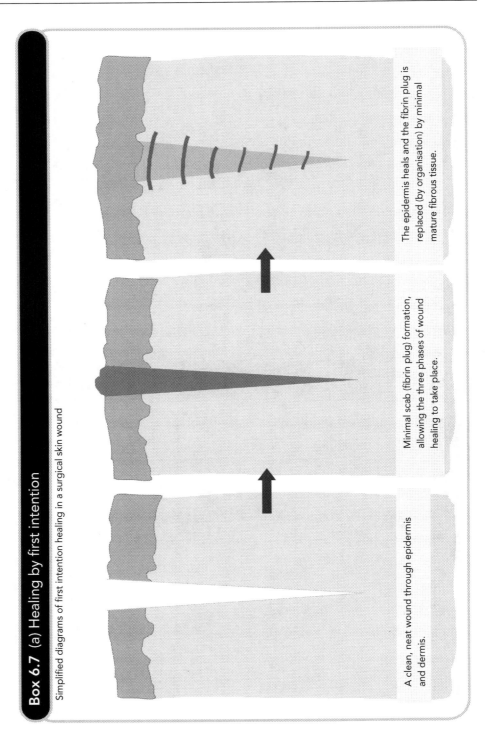

A clean, neat wound through epidermis and dermis.

Minimal scab (fibrin plug) formation, allowing the three phases of wound healing to take place.

The epidermis heals and the fibrin plug is replaced (by organisation) by minimal mature fibrous tissue.

Box 6.7 (Continued) (b) Healing by second intention

Simplified diagrams of second intention healing in a skin wound with a greater loss of tissue than shown in Box 6.7(a).

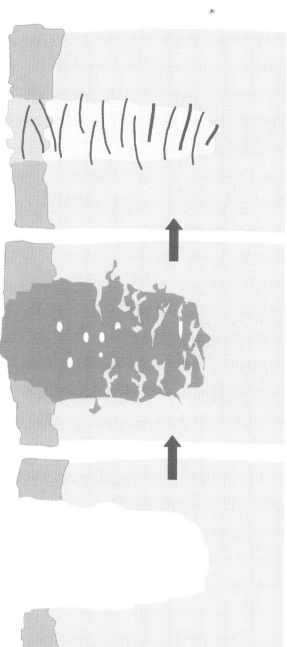

A larger wound involving epidermis and dermis.

More scab (fibrin plug) formation required to fill gap than in Box 6.7(a), which takes longer to organise. Epithelium takes longer to grow over the top and may not manage to grow back completely.

The fibrin plug is replaced (by organisation) by a larger fibrous tissue (scar) than in Box 6.7(a). This scar will contract as it matures. If epithelial re-growth was incomplete, the fibrous scar will extend to the skin surface.

the resulting scar may pucker up or form an indentation, and therefore a less cosmetic result.

Healing in various tissues

What about healing in other tissues apart from skin? Well, the principles we have just discussed in skin still apply, so to illustrate this let us look at a few different organs and see how they tend to heal.

Liver

Liver has excellent powers of regeneration provided damage is not too extensive or chronic. In the case of chronic or extensive damage to the liver both regeneration and organisation occur, so there will be mitotic division of functional liver cells plus some scarring.

There is a specific condition of the liver in aged dogs called *nodular liver regeneration*. This condition has an uncertain cause, possibly involving a toxin, but it seems that there is ongoing liver damage with focal (nodules) of regeneration and intervening scar tissue so that eventually the liver can resemble a large bunch of grapes.

Kidney and lungs

These tissues have some regenerative ability if the injury is not too extensive and the supporting connective tissues remain intact. Usually, there is incomplete regeneration and healing by organisation (scarring).

Heart

Heart muscle cells can hypertrophy but are not able to regenerate if neighbouring cells are irreversibly damaged, so the heart tends to heal by organisation (scarring). Areas of fibrous scarring are not able to contract; a scarred heart (after bouts of damage such as ischaemia, see Chapter 6) therefore may be less efficient at contracting and pumping blood.

Nervous system

- *Peripheral nervous system*: Regrowth of parts of surviving nerves is possible, so in time an area may regain at least part, if not all, of its nerve supply.

- *Central nervous system*: In the central nervous system (brain and spinal cord) there is very limited ability to regenerate damaged nerves. Note that this is a very active area of research, so repair of spinal injuries may, in time, become possible with treatment.

Healing regulation and control

Protein growth factors (produced by inflammatory cells) stimulate and control events. Local factors are also important, such as stimulatory factors from damaged tissue, or the quality of the blood supply. Inhibitory as well as stimulatory factors are involved to allow remodelling, and to stop healing processes when required – that is, when adequate healing has been achieved.

What can impair, prevent or alter healing?

- *Severe prolonged damage*: In which there has been loss of the connective tissue framework or too many of the cells have been damaged to be able to regenerate the tissue (or they are permanent cells unable to regenerate anyway). These conditions tend to favour repair by fibrosis (scarring) rather than regeneration.
- *Contamination*: Presence of large amounts of exudate, dirt, bacteria and/or necrotic tissue tend to prolong the inflammatory phase and delay healing.
- *Inadequate blood supply*: A good blood supply is required for successful healing.
- *Systemic hormonal disorders*: Such as diabetes mellitus and hyperadrenocorticism tend to alter metabolism and activity of the cells involved.
- *Inadequate nutrition*: Protein and energy are particularly important for healing.
- *Movement*: Such as inadequate immobilisation of a healing limb tends to allow wound edges to move against each other and this impairs healing.
- *Self-trauma*: Licking, biting, scratching of wounded areas may allow bacterial contamination or irritation, which prolongs inflammation and slows healing.
- *Old age*: Later in life, blood circulation may be poorer and state of nutrition more variable. Fibrous tissue may proliferate (organisation) but regeneration is impaired.
- *Immunodeficiency diseases*: Immune cells are important in directing the inflammatory phase. Impaired immune function may also allow bacterial contaminants to survive.

- *Chemotherapeutic drugs* and *radiation*: Have detrimental effects on many actively dividing cells, including the cells important in healing.
- *Denervation* (loss of, or damage to, nerves): Alters movement of limbs (possibly allowing more movement of wound edges), decreases blood supply to area, and may encourage self-trauma since there will be reduced pain sensation in the affected area.

Proud flesh

Equine nurses in particular may encounter an aberrant type of healing, usually on horses' legs, which is known as 'proud' flesh. Proud flesh is excess granulation tissue that forms a domed area protruding from or standing 'proud' of the adjacent skin level. Proud flesh can form where epithelial regeneration is slower or less effective than healing in the underlying tissues. The underlying tissues granulate more quickly and since they do not have the overlying epidermis to guide them this granulation tissue just goes on forming. Proud flesh can be cut away surgically but will simply reform unless there is an overlying epithelial layer to keep it in check. Artificial epidermis or skin grafts may be used in horses with proud flesh, to control and direct proper wound healing.

Summary of key points in Chapter 6

- How tissues repair or heal after injury depend on the ability of the cells making up that tissue to regenerate themselves (i.e. whether they are labile, stable or permanent cells).
- Tissues repair or heal by the processes of regeneration and organisation; both processes tend to occur in most tissues. In areas with less ability to heal by regeneration (more permanent cells), more organisation will occur and scars are more likely to form. Scars are non-functional, but tough, fibrous tissue.
- In superficial (epithelial) wounds, the epidermis readily regenerates under a protective serum crust. In deeper wounds, the regeneration of the epidermis acts as a guide and protector for the underlying tissues, which tend to repair by organisation.
- The amount of organisation required to fill a wound is related to the degree of scar formation (fibrosis). Simple clean wounds heal by first intention (primary union) with little scarring. More extensive or contaminated wounds heal by second intention (secondary union) with more marked scar formation.

Test yourself questions on Chapter 6

1. In healing of tissue, the extent to which the new tissue is the same as the tissue that was previously there depends on which two factors?

2. What is meant by regeneration of tissue? Write briefly how it differs from organisation.

3. Name the three phases of organisation, and write brief notes about what occurs in each stage.

4. Describe healing in a skin wound where there has been relatively superficial epithelial (epidermal) damage only.

5. Building on your answer to question 4, briefly discuss healing of a clean, incised (surgical) skin wound (i.e. which extends through the epidermis and into the dermis below). How would this differ in an irregular, non-surgical wound which again involves both epidermis and dermis?

6. Give four factors which may impair, prevent or alter healing in domestic animals.

Chapter 7

Circulatory Disorders

The normal circulatory system

Special note regarding capillaries
Lymphoid circulation
How does interstitial fluid gather in the tissues?

Oedema

Types of oedema (see Box 7.5)
Distribution of oedema

Impaired blood supply to tissues

Ischaemia
Infarction

Clotting (coagulation) of blood

Disseminated intravascular coagulation
Haemorrhage (or *hemorrhage*)
Thrombosis
Embolism

Shock

Pathological effects of shock

Aims of Chapter 7

- To define the main disorders of the circulatory system relating to tissue perfusion and blood clotting, namely, oedema, ischaemia, infarction, haemorrhage, thrombosis, embolism and shock
- To understand the pathogenesis of these conditions and their pathological effects on the body

The normal circulatory system

In this chapter, reference will be made to terms and processes, such as necrosis and inflammation that we discussed in earlier chapters. You might find it useful to ensure you refer back to these topics as you read this chapter – that will help to link the areas together more completely in your mind.

First, some revision. It is worth reminding ourselves a few basic facts about the blood circulatory system in animals. Think about the following questions – cover up the answers and test yourself:

- *What are the functions of the (blood) circulatory system in animals?*
  - *Transport of blood constituents* such as O_2, nutrients, salts, waste products (e.g. CO_2 and urea), hormones and chemical messengers (called *mediators*)
  - *Regulation of body temperature* conserving heat for vital areas by constriction of capillaries in non-vital parts, like the skin. Transporting warm blood to the skin and dilating the capillaries to help cool the body down
  - *Defences against diseases* – inflammatory cells and inflammatory mediators
  - *Fluid regulation* – water, salts and proteins
  - *Blood clotting mechanisms* – platelets and proteins to slow or stop bleeding
- *What are the components of blood in animals?*
  - Red cells
  - White cells
  - Platelets
  - Water
  - Plasma proteins
  - Salts
  - Other:

- Hormones, enzymes, inflammatory mediators, antibodies and growth factors
- Potentially also – pharmacological substances (treatments, anaesthetics and preventative drugs), pathogens (infectious agents), toxins and neoplastic cells

- *What are the components of the circulatory system itself?* (see Box 7.1)

Special note regarding capillaries

Capillaries are very small fine vessels – there are very many miles of capillaries in the body. They are so small and yet so important because their total volume means that all together they can contain a huge amount of blood.

Here are a few important facts about capillaries:

- Capillaries form fine *capillary beds* which are situated between the arterial flow (blood from the heart) and the venous flow (blood returning to the heart).
- The amount and speed of blood flow in these areas is affected by various influences.
- All vessels are lined by a layer of flat cells called *endothelial cells* which form the inner *endothelium*. Whereas bigger vessels have outer layers of smooth muscle and connective tissue around the endothelium, capillaries lack this extra structure to their wall. Capillary walls are not much more than a single-layered crazy paving of endothelial cells (Box 7.2). Endothelial cells secrete a substance called a *glycoprotein*. This glycoprotein has some important actions, which are particularly vital in capillaries:
  - Glycoprotein prevents blood clotting – so that normal healthy capillaries do not clog up with blood clots, which would be catastrophic for the animal's blood circulation.
  - Glycoprotein protects intercellular junctions – these are the joins between endothelial cells (the gaps between the crazy paving tiles – see Box 7.2).
- Capillaries are normally slightly leaky and there is a small net outflow of fluid from capillaries into surrounding tissues, and then it becomes known as *interstitial fluid*. Interstitial fluid bathes the cells and tissues but is 'outside' of the blood vessels. Fortunately, otherwise we would keep swelling up with fluid in our tissues and our blood circulation would run out of fluid, the *lymph vessels* are able to gather up this excess fluid and return it to the blood circulation (see section *lymphoid circulation* on page 120).

Box 7.1 The components of the blood circulatory system

Heart: The heart is divided into left and right sides, and into four chambers – the left and right atria and the left and right ventricles.

The atria are smaller and their walls are not as muscular as the ventricles. Blood from the body enters the right ventricle; blood from the lungs enters the left ventricle.

Blood then passes into the more muscular ventricles and is pumped (by the contraction of the heart muscle) to the body from the left ventricle (the start of the systemic circulation) and to the lungs from the right ventricle (the start of the pulmonary circulation). The left ventricle is the most muscular chamber because the blood from this chamber has further to go.

There are valves between the atria and the ventricles which make sure all the blood passes to the ventricles and does not flow back into the atria again.

The blood to the body is freshly oxygenated because it has just returned to the heart from the lungs. The blood to the lungs has just returned from the body and is low in oxygen and high in carbon dioxide.

Arteries: The arteries are the blood vessels which carry blood from the heart to either the body or the lungs. The main artery from the left side of the heart is the aorta, the main artery from the right side of the heart is called the pulmonary artery. The main arteries divide to produce smaller ones, and so on. The smallest arteries are called arterioles. Arterioles lead into the smallest vessels called capillaries (see below). Arteries have thick muscular walls because they operate at high pressure and they transmit the beat of the heart muscle (which can be felt as the pulse). This is why damage to arteries – especially the larger ones – is very serious. They bleed in high pressure spurts and arterial 'bleeds' can be difficult to stop simply by applying pressure.

Veins: The veins carry blood back to the heart. The main vein to the left side of the heart is the vena cava, the main vein to the right side of the heart is the pulmonary vein. There are smaller vessels in the venous system called venules (similar to the arterioles in the arterial system). Veins have thinner walls and they are usually at less pressure. Venous 'bleeds' do not spurt and many can be stopped by applying pressure to the damaged vessel as this encourages blood clotting.

Capillaries: In the tissues, whether the lungs or the tissues of the body, there are very thin-walled vessels called capillaries, which form fine meshes called capillary beds. The capillary beds ensure maximum contact between blood and tissues and allow gas exchange (see text and Boxes 7.2). The blood vessels entering the capillary bed are known as the *arterial supply*; the blood vessels leaving the capillary bed are known as the *venous supply*.

There is another circulatory network called the lymphatic circulation which drains fluid from the tissues, which has leaked out from the blood back into the blood circulatory system (see text and Box 7.3).

The following diagram is a summary of the main parts of the blood circulatory system (the lymphatic system is omitted for simplicity but is dealt with in Box 7.3).

Box 7.1 (*Continued*) The components of the blood circulatory system

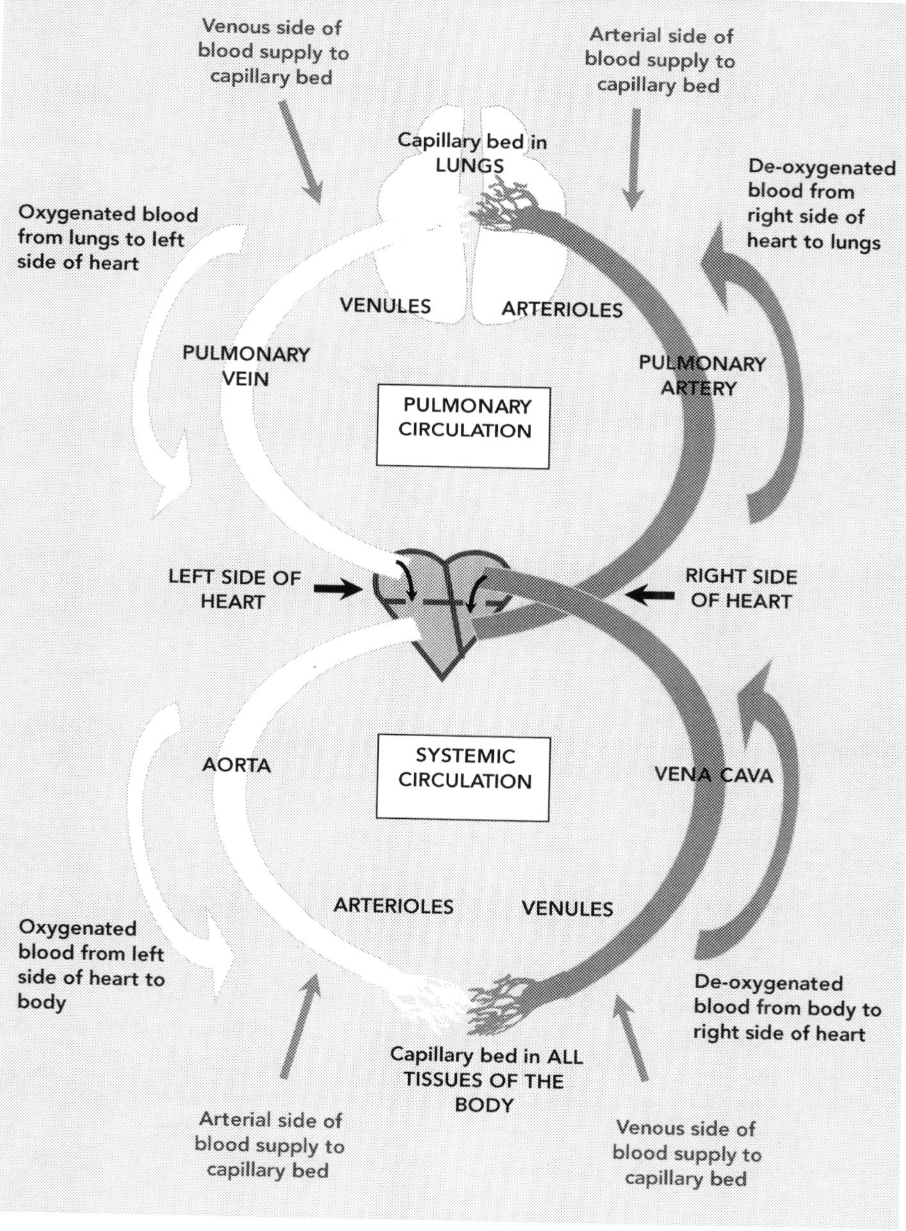

Venous side of
blood supply to
capillary bed

Arterial side of
blood supply to
capillary bed

Capillary bed in
LUNGS

De-oxygenated
blood from
right side of
heart to lungs

Oxygenated blood
from lungs to left
side of heart

VENULES   ARTERIOLES

PULMONARY
VEIN

PULMONARY
ARTERY

PULMONARY
CIRCULATION

LEFT SIDE OF
HEART

RIGHT SIDE
OF HEART

AORTA

SYSTEMIC
CIRCULATION

VENA CAVA

Oxygenated
blood from left
side of heart to
body

ARTERIOLES   VENULES

De-oxygenated
blood from body to
right side of heart

Capillary bed in ALL
TISSUES OF THE
BODY

Arterial side of
blood supply to
capillary bed

Venous side of
blood supply to
capillary bed

Box 7.2 The structure and function of capillaries (Part 1)

As shown in Box 7.1, capillaries form fine *capillary beds* which are situated between the arterial flow (blood from the heart) and the venous flow (blood returning to the heart). The diagram below shows a simplified representation of a capillary bed.

The fine mesh-work of the capillary bed ensures the maximum supply of oxygen and nutrients to the tissues from the blood, and allows waste from the tissues to be removed as efficiently as possible.

Capillary bed

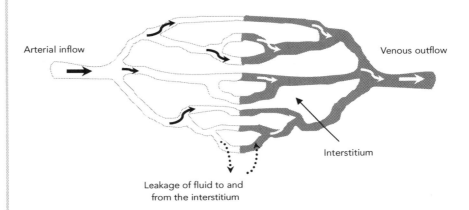

Arterial inflow

Venous outflow

Interstitium

Leakage of fluid to and
from the interstitium

The amount and speed of flow of blood through capillary beds is affected by various factors, which act to open up (dilate) or close (contract) the arterial inflow or venous outflow vessels.

Capillaries are normally leaky and there is an outflow of fluid to and fro from capillaries into surrounding tissues and back again (see dotted arrows in the diagram of the capillary bed above). The fluid contributes to *interstitial fluid* which bathes the cells and tissues, but is outside of the blood vessels (in the virtual space called the interstitium).

There is normally a small net outflow into the interstitium, i.e. slightly more escape of fluid from the capillary bed than is re-absorbed. Fortunately, so that we do not keep swelling up with fluid in our tissues, excess fluid is gathered up by the *lymph vessels* and drained back into the blood circulation (see *lymphoid circulation*, text and Box 7.3).

Box 7.2 (*Continued*) The structure and function of capillaries (Part 2)

All blood vessels are lined by a layer of slender cells called *endothelial cells* which together make up the inner layer of the vessel wall – the *endothelium*.

Endothelial cells secrete an important substance called a *glycoprotein*. Under normal circumstances, glycoprotein:

- acts like a non-stick coating on a saucepan and prevents blood clotting in the vessels
- protects the *intercellular* junctions between endothelial cells (i.e. the gaps between the crazy paving tiles)

In the bigger blood vessels (arteries, veins, arterioles and venules) the endothelium is supported by outer layers of smooth muscle and connective tissue. Capillaries do not have this extra structure to their walls, so in effect capillary walls are formed from not much more than a thin-layered 'crazy paving' of endothelial cells

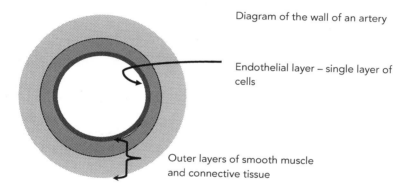

Diagram of the wall of an artery

Endothelial layer – single layer of cells

Outer layers of smooth muscle and connective tissue

Veins are thinner walled than arteries, as they are under less pressure, but they are still more substantial than capillaries – see below.

Diagram of a capillary – the wall is composed of a single layer of endothelial cells

Note that these two diagrams are not to the same scale – arteries are much, much bigger than capillaries!

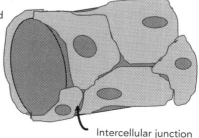

Intercellular junction

Lymphoid circulation

Lymph vessels gather up fluid called *interstitial fluid* from the tissues (*interstitium*) and return it to the blood vascular system. (This fluid is called *lymph* when it is in the lymphoid circulation (see Box 7.3).)

Lymph vessels are thinner walled and are at lower pressure than blood vessels. Like blood vessels they are of various sizes, starting small (like capillaries) and getting gradually larger as they drain back towards the blood circulatory system. They have lymph nodes at intervals along them, which act as filters and are important in the function of the immune system.

Box 7.3 The lymphoid circulation

As discussed in Box 7.2, capillaries are leaky and there is an outflow of fluid to the surrounding tissues and back again. The fluid which leaves the capillaries contributes to *interstitial fluid*, bathing the cells and tissues and allowing nutrient delivery, gas exchange and removal of waste products from the cells.

There is normally a small net outflow of fluid into the interstitium – that is fluid lost from the circulation in the tissues slightly exceeds the amount re-absorbed. Normally, to prevent us swelling up due to accumulated fluid in our tissues, the excess interstitial fluid is collected by the *lymph vessels* and drained back into the blood circulation (pale grey dotted arrows in diagram below). The fluid in the lymphoid circulation is called *lymph*.

Lymph vessels are thinner walled and are at lower pressure than blood vessels. Like blood vessels they are of various sizes, starting small (like capillaries) and getting gradually larger as they drain back towards the blood circulatory system. They have lymph nodes at intervals along them, which act as filters and are important in the function of the immune system. (Lymph nodes can also inadvertently filter neoplastic cells, as we discuss in Chapter 8.)

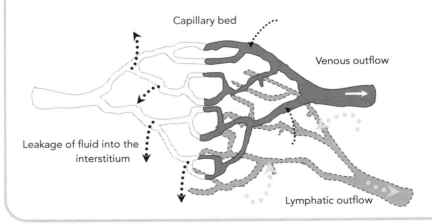

Box 7.3 (*Continued*) The lymphoid circulation

The exact position of the vessel draining lymph into the blood circulatory system varies slightly between species but it is usually somewhere near to the right atrium.

Diagram of the lymph circulation – the lymph is drained back to the blood circulatory system near to the right atrium

For simplicity, the arterial side of the circulation is not shown. In addition, note that the pulmonary circulation is not shown, but lymph vessels also drain the interstitial tissue around capillary beds in the lungs.

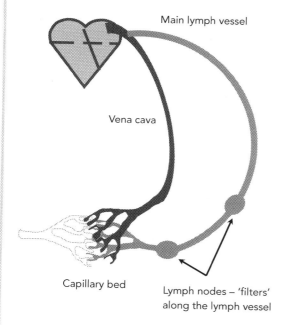

Main lymph vessel

Vena cava

Capillary bed

Lymph nodes – 'filters' along the lymph vessel

Animals with increased outflow of fluid from the blood circulation, or with decreased drainage of lymph accumulate interstitial fluid, and this is called *oedema* (see text).

The lymph drains back into the blood circulation near to the right side of the heart. The exact position of the vessel draining lymph into the blood varies slightly between species.

How does interstitial fluid gather in the tissues?

There are two forces which affect the pressure of fluid within the circulation (see Box 7.4):

- *Hydrostatic pressure* is the pressure of fluid in blood vessels. Think of the pressure that builds up in a hosepipe when you turn on the tap. The walls of the hose become tense as the pressure of the water builds up and if you do not steady the free end of the hose, the water (hydrostatic) pressure makes the hose whip round like an angry snake. The hydrostatic pressure of the blood normally tends to push fluid out into the interstitium from the (leaky) capillaries.
- *Osmotic pressure* is the pressure that develops due to differences in the concentration of substances dissolved in fluid (solutes) separated by a slightly leaky membrane (such as a capillary wall). If two solutions, one concentrated and one dilute, are separated by a leaky membrane, the water will tend to flow into the more concentrated side in order to even up (equilibrate) the concentrations of the two solutions. We say that the solute that is acting to draw water through the leaky membrane is *osmotically active*. In the body, solutes exerting osmotic pressure include *salts* (such as sodium chloride) and, especially important in the blood, *plasma proteins*. We noted above that capillary walls are normally slightly leaky. Large molecules, like proteins in blood (plasma proteins), however, are not normally able to pass across the leaky capillary walls as they are too big. This means that they are usually retained within the blood circulation and exert osmotic pressure, tending to draw fluid *from* the interstitium and into the blood. Though, as noted above, in a healthy individual there is *normally a slight net loss of fluid from blood into the interstitium*.

Oedema

Oedema (or edema in American texts) is the accumulation of excessive amounts of interstitial fluid. Oedema fluid causes a soft swelling of the tissue, which characteristically can be 'pitted' – this means that you can press into the surface of oedematous tissue with your finger or an instrument and leave an indentation. (Conversely, swelling due to, for instance, a soft tumour will not 'pit' when pressed.)

There are different types of oedema depending on how the fluid accumulation has been caused. In all of these types of oedema, the lymphatic circulation is not able to remove adequately the excess fluid from the tissues.

Types of oedema (see Box 7.5)

- *Inflammatory oedema* occurs when there is a site of inflammation in the body. Inflammation often leads to damage to the

Box 7.4 Hydrostatic and osmotic pressure

Hydrostatic pressure = the fluid pressure in blood vessels. The hydrostatic pressure of the blood normally tends to push fluid out into the interstitium from the leaky capillaries.

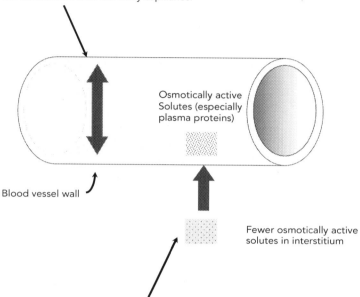

Osmotically active Solutes (especially plasma proteins)

Blood vessel wall

Fewer osmotically active solutes in interstitium

Osmotic pressure = the pressure that develops due to differences in the concentration of substances (solutes) dissolved in fluids either side of a slightly leaky membrane (such as a capillary wall). If two solutions, one concentrated and one dilute, are separated by a leaky membrane, the water will tend to flow into the more concentrated side until the concentrations of the two solutions are evened up (equilibrated). We say that the solute that is acting to draw water through the leaky membrane is *osmotically active*. In the body, solutes exerting osmotic pressure include *salts* (such as sodium chloride) and, especially important in the blood, *plasma proteins*.

Note that there are osmotically active substances in the interstitium and so there will be an osmotic pull from the blood *into* the interstitium as well, tending to equilibrate the solutions either side of the vessel wall.

In a healthy individual there is *normally a slight net loss of fluid from blood into the interstitium.*

Box 7.5 Summary of types of oedema

Think about the ways these types of oedema develop, you should be able to follow the process through.

Type of oedema	Fluid characteristic	How does it develop?	Why does it develop?
Inflammatory	High protein Contains cells (cellular)	Leaky capillaries	Damage to endothelial wall
Non-inflammatory	Low protein	↑ plasma hydrostatic pressure	↑ venous pressure due to heart disease; ↓ venous outflow (blockage – neoplasia, fibrosis/scars and trauma)
		↓ plasma osmotic pressure	e.g. loss of plasma protein (malnutrition, chronic diarrhoea); renal disease; ↓ synthesis of plasma protein (chronic liver disease); anaemia
		↑ tissue osmotic pressure	↑ salt and water retention (kidney disease)
		↓ lymph drainage	Lymphatic obstruction (blockage – neoplasia, fibrosis/scars and trauma)

endothelial lining of the capillaries, meaning that they become more leaky than normal, allowing even large molecules like plasma proteins to move out into the interstitium. You will remember from the discussion above that large molecules, like plasma proteins, exert osmotic pressure, therefore when they escape into the interstitium they attract fluid out from the blood too. The plasma proteins do not enter the lymphatic circulation but hang around in the tissues keeping much of the accumulated fluid with them.

Inflammatory oedema characteristically is high in protein content and may be very cellular as it contains white cells attracted to the site of inflammation (see Chapter 4).

- *Non-inflammatory oedema* has a number of causes, discussed below. The endothelial lining of the capillaries more often remains intact in non-inflammatory oedema, so this form of oedema fluid tends to be low in protein and usually does not contain cells.

Causes of non-inflammatory oedema

- *Increased blood (plasma) hydrostatic pressure*: Increased hydrostatic pressure may happen for a number of reasons (see next paragraph) but however it occurs, the increased pressure in the circulation pushes fluid out into the interstitium.

  How could this increase in hydrostatic pressure occur? It occurs because of an increase in pressure in the venous circulation, in other words, on the 'return to heart side' of the capillary bed. This may be due to a simple blockage, not allowing blood to pass back to the heart (e.g. a tumour, or scar tissue, or pressure from a constricting bandage for instance) or there could be heart disease in which case the heart cannot pump blood onwards into the arteries, causing a back-pressure in the venous circulation.

- *Decreased plasma osmotic pressure*: If the osmotic pressure of the blood plasma is decreased the blood loses its ability to retain fluid osmotically. This decrease in osmotic pressure may happen if there is loss of plasma protein, such as in malnutrition or in chronic diarrhoea or renal disease. Osmotic pressure may decrease if plasma protein is not produced in adequate quantities, such as in chronic liver disease. Finally, chronic anaemia may cause a decrease in plasma osmotic pressure.

- *Increased tissue osmotic pressure*: Osmotic pressure works both ways across the blood vessel walls since the interstitial fluid exerts its own osmotic pressure. If the osmotic pressure of the interstitium is increased, for instance, if there is salt retention due to kidney disease, then the interstitial fluid can draw water from the blood by osmosis. In kidney disease there may be decreased fluid excretion in urine too, further exacerbating the problem.

- *Lymphatic obstruction*: If the lymph drainage system is not working efficiently, perhaps because the lymph vessels are blocked, then the normal small net outflow of fluid from the blood circulation becomes a problem. The fluid accumulates in the interstitium and is not removed by the lymph vessels. Such a blockage may happen due to a tumour, or scar tissue, or pressure from a constricting bandage, for instance, or simply due to immobility, since the fluid flow in the low-pressure lymphatic vessels is aided by movement of the limbs. If the nearby veins are also affected by the same constrictions as the lymphatic vessels then the problem is even worse. (Note arteries and arterioles are harder to constrict because they have thick muscular walls, whereas veins, venules and lymphatic vessels have thinner collapsible walls.)

Distribution of oedema

Oedema may form in different ways and to different extents, depending on the cause.

- *Localised oedema*: One area affected, such as oedema caused by an area of inflammation or a local blockage of venous or lymph flow, e.g. tight bandage or plaster cast on a limb.
- *Generalised oedema*: This is widespread and more likely to be caused by diffuse problems with venous drainage (e.g. heart disease) or general decrease in osmotic pressure (loss of plasma protein due to chronic diarrhoea).
- *Dependent oedema*: This is when gravity tends to lead to pooling of the fluid on ventral areas or lower points of the body. For instance, dependent oedema may happen along the ventral chest or around the lower part of the legs.
- *Oedema in specific locations*: Oedema may be assigned a particular name and you may hear about *hydrothorax* (accumulation of fluid inside the thoracic cavity of the chest); *hydropericardium* (accumulation of fluid inside the pericardial sac around the heart); and *ascites* (accumulation of fluid inside the peritoneal cavity of the abdomen).
- *Anasarca*: This is diffuse marked accumulation of fluid just under the skin (subcutaneous fluid) and it may happen as a result of chronic heart failure, though dead baby animals may occasionally be found to be *anasarcous* at the time of birth and the mothers are then unable to give birth to them naturally, and require a caesarean section.

In most instances oedema is an indication of something else going wrong in the body (e.g. heart disease) but it may not necessarily be harmful in itself. There are some situations, however, when oedema itself may be damaging and even life-threatening.

When may oedema be life-threatening?

Think about what oedema is – an accumulation of fluid. In certain circumstances this will be particularly damaging, such as:

- *Pulmonary oedema*: Accumulation of fluid in the lungs. This is what happens in chronic heart disease. If not treated, the fluid builds up and affects the function of the lungs causing breathlessness and coughing.
- *Brain*: The brain is encased in a rigid container, the skull, so if swelling due to oedema of the brain (cerebral oedema) occurs, the brain presses against the skull and serious brain impairment may result, leading to headaches, loss of consciousness and slowed breathing. This can happen in a condition known as salt poisoning,

when animals (such as pigs) have inadequate access to water and are eating relatively salty rations.

- *Larynx*: Accumulation of fluid in the throat, for instance, when an animal catches a bee and is stung. The venom in the sting damages endothelial cells and makes the blood vessels leaky so that oedema accumulates in the mouth and throat and this can stop the animal's breathing.

Impaired blood supply to tissues

Two terms are used in pathology in relation to decreased blood supply to tissues, these are:

- *Ischaemia* (or ischemia) which is decreased blood flow or *perfusion* and therefore decreased supply of vital nutrients, especially oxygen, to that area.
- *Infarction* means death (necrosis) of the area of tissue as a result of ischaemia.

Both these terms are discussed in more detail in the next sections.

Ischaemia

This is pronounced *is-kee-mia* and comes from the Greek words '*is-chein*' meaning 'to hold back' and '*haemo*' which refers to blood. So literally, ischaemia means preventing blood from flowing into the tissue.

The effects on the tissue of a period of reduced blood supply can be reversible, in other words, tissue damage either will not result from a period of ischaemia or it will occur but will not be permanent (i.e. the tissue heals), but this depends on:

- The duration of the period of ischaemia: Tissue damage resulting from a short period of ischaemia is more likely to be reversible than extended periods of ischaemia.
- The metabolic demands of the tissue: An organ with a low metabolic rate and therefore low requirements of vital nutrients and oxygen is less likely to be damaged by a period of ischaemia.

Causes of ischaemia
See Box 7.6 for common causes of ischaemia.

Infarction

Infarction is the death (*necrosis*) of tissue as result of ischaemia. An *infarct* is an area of ischaemic necrosis in a tissue or organ (Box 7.7), so in this case the period of ischaemia has had permanent effects.

Box 7.6 Common causes of ischaemia

Thrombosis   **Embolism**   **Vasoconstriction**

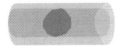      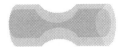

Intravascular coagulation   Mass of any material   Spasm in wall of vessel,
(blood clotting within   travelling in blood and   various causes
blood vessels of a living   able to lodge in vessels
animal – not the same as
blood clotting as a
response to vessel
damage)

Compression   **Vasculitis**   **Vessel damage**

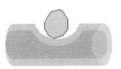   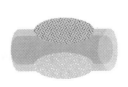   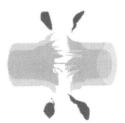

For example, due to a   Inflammation of the   Vessels torn by a bad
tumour growing next to   vessel wall   wound or bone fracture
vessel,
or a tight bandage

Box 7.7 Infarction

Infarction is defined as death (by *necrosis*) of tissue as result of ischaemia (loss of blood supply).

An *infarct* is an area of necrosis due to ischaemia (or *ischaemic necrosis*) in a tissue or organ.

Usually, it is the arterial supply that is affected in some way to cause *arterial infarction* of the affected tissue; venous infarction does occur though it is less common.

The diagram below represents a block of cells, to which the arterial blood supply has been drastically reduced for some reason – in this case it looks like there is a *thrombus* blocking an arteriole. The artery affected is a smaller branch towards the end of the arterial supply so a focal infarct has resulted – that is, a well-defined area of necrosis has developed as a result.

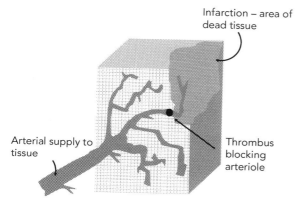

Infarction – area of dead tissue

Arterial supply to tissue

Thrombus blocking arteriole

The diagram below represents as *global infarction*; there is blockage of a large or proximal artery (an artery nearer to the heart) which is responsible for supplying blood to wider area. In this case there is more severe or extensive infarction of the tissue.

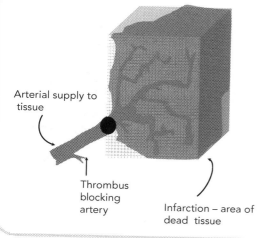

Arterial supply to tissue

Thrombus blocking artery

Infarction – area of dead tissue

Usually, the arterial supply is compromised in some way causing arterial infarction of a tissue; less commonly, venous infarction occurs.

The extent of infarction (that is the extent of necrosis in a tissue) depends on:

- the level of the vessel blocked and
- the presence of an alternative blood supply (see below in the section *Which organs are most sensitive to ischaemia?*)

So, for instance, a *focal infarction* would result from blockage of a small or terminal artery. Examples of focal infarction would include:

- blockage of an artery in the kidney cortex
- blockage of an artery or arteriole in the heart causing myocardial infarction
- intestinal infarct, such as that occasionally caused by roundworm (Strongyle) infection in horses

Global infarction, on the other hand, occurs when there is blockage of a large or proximal artery (artery nearer the heart) which is responsible for supplying blood to a wider area of the organ or tissue; in this case, there will be more severe or extensive infarction of the tissue. For instance, an entire lung lobe may be infarcted due to torsion of the lobe (twisting of the lobe causing blockage of the arterial supply to that lobe).

Progression of an infarct

When irreversible ischaemia occurs and the affected tissue starts to die there are recognisable stages of development of the resulting infarct. (See Box 7.8. You may also find it helpful to refer back to the section on tissue healing in Chapter 6.)

- An area of pale tissue (*pallor*) will be visible from approximately 24 hours after the blood supply has been interrupted. The pale area will correspond to the area of tissue normally supplied by the now impaired blood vessel. This early infarct will be surrounded by a zone of *inflammation* (an inflammatory border).
- *Healing by regeneration or organisation* of the area (see *tissue healing*, Chapter 6).
- Organisation (if tissue is not able to regenerate) will mean that scar tissue will form (see *tissue healing*, Chapter 6). In the final stage the *scar contracts*. This contraction is responsible for the hard shrunken nature of old established infarcts, for instance, the kidneys of old cats with chronic infarcts are nodular, small and firm.

Box 7.8 Progression of an infarct

When an infarct starts to develop due to ischaemia in a tissue there are recognisable stages of development.

Pallor (paleness) – visible from approximately 24 hours after the blood supply has been interrupted. The paleness occurs in the area of tissue normally supplied by the now impaired blood vessel. This early infarct will be surrounded by a zone of *inflammation* (an inflammatory border).

The following diagram builds on the simplified version in Box 7.6 to illustrate these changes.

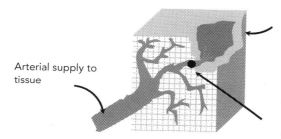

Infarction – area of dead tissue. Appears pale with a peripheral zone of inflammation.

Arterial supply to tissue

Thrombus blocking arteriole

If tissue is not able to regenerate, then organisation of the area follows (see Chapter 6).

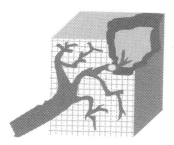

Organisation of infarcted area – formation of immature fibrous tissue.

Fibrous scar forms in area of organised tissue. In the final stage the scar contracts, which is responsible for the hard shrunken nature of old established infarcts.

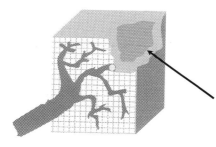

Old established infarction. Mature fibrous tissue has developed which has contracted and formed a hard scar, which deforms the tissue in this area.

Which organs are most sensitive to ischaemia (and therefore to infarction – death of tissue)?

Organs or tissues whose cells are very sensitive to decreased oxygen supply (hypoxia) are likely to be most harmed by ischaemia. Examples of such sensitive tissues are brain, kidney and heart.

Which organs are less sensitive to ischaemia?

Tissues less sensitive to ischaemia are mainly those with more than one blood supply, so if one is diminished, vital nutrients and oxygen can be supplied by other vessels, e.g. lung, liver, muscle and intestine.

We now move on from impaired blood supply to discuss the important process of blood clotting, and then to learn about what can go wrong to alter normal blood clotting.

Clotting (coagulation) of blood

Blood clotting (coagulation) depends to a large extent on conversion of a soluble protein in the blood called *fibrinogen* to the insoluble protein *fibrin*. Strands of fibrin are an important part of the structure of a blood clot. Formation of fibrin is brought about by a chain reaction or cascade of enzymes in the blood. These enzymes are called *clotting factors* and they are produced as an inactive form by the liver. The inactive form of each factor is activated in sequence during the clotting cascade, each newly formed active factor then activates the next factor in the chain (this is a similar arrangement to the complement cascade of proteins of the immune response – see Chapter 5). Several steps in this cascade also require calcium and several require vitamin K, to help the reactions to occur.

You may see reference in other texts to two initial pathways of clotting factor activation called the *extrinsic* and *intrinsic* pathways, which are triggered by slightly different things, but the final part of the process is the same – the conversion of fibrinogen to fibrin. Further details of the coagulation cascade may be found in other pathology textbooks, especially those dealing with clinical pathology. The process is summarised in Box 7.9.

So, fibrin is the fibrous protein part of a blood clot but particles called *platelets* are also an important part of the clotting process. Box 7.10 discusses a few features of platelets before going onto describe blood coagulation in more detail.

There are a number of triggers for the coagulation process, such as damage to blood vessel walls which exposes the blood to collagen underlying the damaged endothelium, or contact between blood and abnormal surfaces, such as glass (as may happen to a blood smear on a microscope slide or a blood sample in a plain tube without

Box 7.9 Fibrin formation in blood coagulation (see also Box 7.11)

Part of blood clotting (coagulation) depends on conversion of a soluble protein in the blood called *fibrinogen* to an insoluble one called *fibrin*. Strands of fibrin bind particles called *platelets* together to form a blood clot (see Boxes 7.10 and 7.11).

Formation of fibrin is brought about by a chain of enzymes in the blood, called *clotting factors*; these enzymes are produced as an inactive form by the liver. The inactive form of each factor is activated in sequence during the coagulation cascade, each newly formed active factor activating the next factor in the chain (compare the complement cascade of proteins in our discussion of immunology – see Chapter 5).

Several steps in this cascade also require calcium and several require vitamin K to help the reactions occur.

There are two initial pathways of clotting factor activation, called the *extrinsic* and *intrinsic* pathways, which are triggered by slightly different things, but the final part of the process is the same – the conversion of fibrinogen to fibrin.

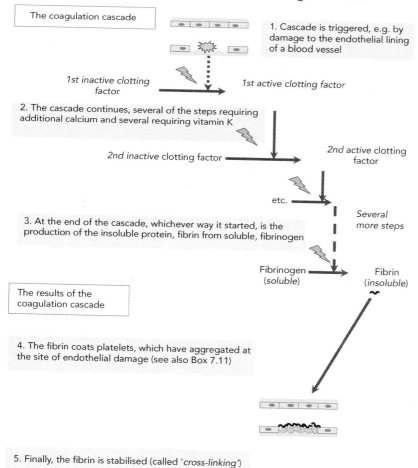

The coagulation cascade

1. Cascade is triggered, e.g. by damage to the endothelial lining of a blood vessel

1st inactive clotting factor → 1st active clotting factor

2. The cascade continues, several of the steps requiring additional calcium and several requiring vitamin K

2nd inactive clotting factor → 2nd active clotting factor

etc.

Several more steps

3. At the end of the cascade, whichever way it started, is the production of the insoluble protein, fibrin from soluble, fibrinogen

Fibrinogen (soluble) → Fibrin (insoluble)

The results of the coagulation cascade

4. The fibrin coats platelets, which have aggregated at the site of endothelial damage (see also Box 7.11)

5. Finally, the fibrin is stabilised (called 'cross-linking')

Box 7.10 A few features of platelets

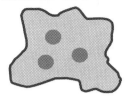

Platelets:
- are flat structures, which contain cytoplasm, other cellular components (organelles) and numerous granules
- are formed in bone marrow from fragmented large cells called *megakaryocytes*
- clump together (*aggregate*) and become *activated* and then *contract* in clotting
- contain granules which, when the platelets are activated, release products that regulate clotting (and that are also actively involved in inflammation and repair)

anti-coagulant). Endothelial cells themselves are also able to initiate the coagulation cascade. To describe the coagulation process in general terms we will discuss what happens when a blood vessel is damaged.

When a vessel is cut or torn, blood starts to escape (haemorrhage) and blood clotting or coagulation is triggered to try to limit, or preferably stop, the blood loss (*haemostasis*). There are recognised stages in the process of coagulation (Box 7.11):

- *Vasoconstriction*: A transient reflex contraction of the smooth muscle in the vessel wall which squeezes the vessel and may help to reduce blood loss. (This blood vessel contraction is not likely to be strong or persistent enough to stop bleeding altogether but it may help to reduce blood loss.)
- *Primary haemostasis*: Injury to the endothelium (from whatever damaged the blood vessel) makes platelets stick to it and become activated.
- *Secondary haemostasis*: The coagulation cascade referred to above is activated by the released contents of the platelet granules resulting in fibrin formation.
- *Clot formation*: Fibrin and platelets clump together at the site of vessel damage to form a solid plug (*clot* or *thrombus*).

Note that there is a system that can counteract the coagulation process. This system is called *fibrinolysis*, literally, '*lysis*' or splitting of fibrin. In the normal circulation a delicate balance is maintained (Box 7.12) – blood needs to be fluid to circulate and to carry out its important transport functions, but equally, it is important that the clotting system is on 'stand by' to plug quickly any leaks in the circulation.

Box 7.11 Clot formation on a vessel wall

The coagulation process can be triggered by various things such as damage to blood vessel walls or contact between blood and abnormal surfaces (such as glass – this happens when normal blood is applied to a microscope slide, for instance).

To illustrate the general features of the coagulation process the following discussion uses the example of damage to a blood vessel wall as the trigger (diagram A).

When a vessel is cut or torn, blood starts to escape (haemorrhage) and blood coagulation (*haemostasis*) is triggered to limit, and preferably stop, the blood loss. There are recognised stages in the process of haemostasis:

Vasoconstriction – a short-term reflex contraction of the smooth muscle in the vessel wall which constricts the vessel to try to reduce blood loss (diagram B). (This blood vessel contraction is not likely to be strong or persistent, so is not enough to stop bleeding altogether).

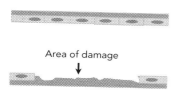

A: Area of damage to vessel, causing loss of endothelial cells and exposure of tissues beneath the endothelial layer.

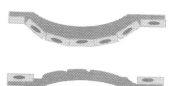

B: Local short-term contraction of smooth muscle of vessel wall.

Primary haemostasis – the exposure of the tissues beneath the endothelium attracts platelets and activates them so that they stick to the area and to each other (diagram C). *Secondary haemostasis* – next, the coagulation cascade of proteins is activated, resulting in fibrin formation. The fibrin and platelets clump together at the site of the damage to form a solid plug (*clot* or *thrombus*) (diagram D).

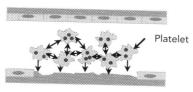

Platelet

C: Platelets clump together on the surface of the exposed sub-endothelial tissues.

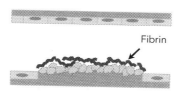

Fibrin

D: The platelets contract and release the contents of their granules which help to promote the coagulation cascade; fibrin is produced.

Box 7.12 The delicate balance of coagulation and fibrinolysis in the blood vascular system

In order to carry out its transport functions, blood obviously needs to be fluid to circulate freely so blood clotting in the blood vessels is not desirable under normal circumstances. On the other hand, it is important that there is also a system to quickly plug any leaks in the circulation to prevent escape of blood, so a clotting system must be on 'stand by' to do this. For normal functioning of the circulatory system a delicate balance has to exist between these two activities.

The latter 'leak-plugging' system is served by the coagulation system (see earlier). The system which counteracts coagulation is called *fibrinolysis* (literally '*lysis*' or splitting of fibrin).

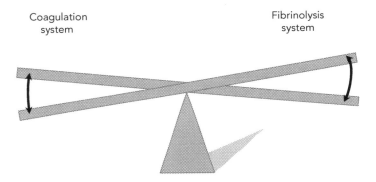

Coagulation system

Fibrinolysis system

A delicate balance exists between the coagulation and fibrinolysis systems in the normal circulation.

Remember that blood clotting and fibrinolysis are normal physiological processes, but that derangements or extremes of either process may shift this balance in favour of one or other of these functions. The result of inappropriate clotting or tendency to haemorrhage could be harmful, or even fatal, for the animal.

There is therefore the potential for clotting to be triggered in undamaged vessels, which would be disastrous for the animal. To stop this happening, clot formation is kept in check (by *fibrinolysis*).

Remember that blood clotting and fibrinolysis are normal physiological processes, but that derangements or extremes of either process may be harmful or even fatal for the animal.

Disseminated intravascular coagulation

A specific disorder of clotting is *disseminated intravascular coagulation* (DIC). This is a very serious condition involving blood clots forming all over the body. DIC is caused by widespread damage to the endothelium of blood vessels in all parts of the body. This damage may be caused by toxins in the bloodstream such as those generated in severe infections. There is diffuse endothelial necrosis because of the toxic damage and this triggers formation of blood clots all over the body. In response to this there is then excess triggering of fibrinolysis to try to break down the clots.

The consequences of DIC include marked depletion of clotting factors (called a *consumption coagulopathy*, because clotting factors are said to be consumed or used up). As a result there will be multiple small haemorrhages all over the body. Although the individual haemorrhages are often small, they are so numerous and widespread that they represent a huge loss of circulating blood volume (see section *Shock* on page 145). The large number of clots which are not broken down effectively will also cause widespread infarction in many tissues and organs. As you may appreciate, development of DIC is a very poor sign for the animal.

Haemorrhage (or *hemorrhage*)

Haemorrhage is used to denote blood loss from the circulatory system.

Causes of haemorrhage
- Blood vessel damage, e.g. trauma (RTA, bone fracture and spleen rupture).
- Ulceration of body surfaces – such as stomach or skin ulcers – which is deep enough to erode an underlying vessel. Ulcers may be caused by chemicals, infectious agents, inflammation, invasive tumours or ischaemic necrosis.
- Rupture of a tumour – many tumours (or neoplasms) have good blood supplies (in Chapter 8, we shall discuss this aspect in more detail, specifically in the section on *angiogenesis*) and may be associated with extensive blood loss if they rupture or ulcerate.

- Haemorrhages can also occur when there is a shift of the delicate clot/fibrinolysis balance in favour of bleeding. This is what happens in disorders called *coagulopathies*.

Coagulopathies
Coagulopathies are disorders of the coagulation mechanism that result from deficiency or infectiveness of any stage of the clotting process. Coagulopathies are described as being *acquired* or *congenital*. Some coagulopathies may be undetected, until unexpected, possibly severe bleeding occurs after minor surgery or after a modest wound. In severe cases the animal may be lame due to bleeding into joints or may pass blood in the faeces. Because of the risk of previously undetected coagulopathy, coagulation tests are often carried out on animals prior to surgery to assess clotting function.

- *Acquired coagulopathies*: This may accompany other severe diseases and may be caused by transient reduction in production, or excessive use (*consumption*), of clotting factors (see DIC above).
  - *Liver disease*: The liver is normally an important site of clotting factor production, aided by vitamin K. Recall that this vitamin is important in several steps of the coagulation cascade. Liver disease therefore has the potential to decrease clotting.
  - *Rodenticides* (rat or mouse poisons): Anti-coagulating rat poisons (e.g. dicoumarol known as Warfarin) act by inhibiting the liver enzymes which are responsible for synthesis of several clotting factors.
  - *Vitamin K deficiency*: Vitamin K is important in the synthesis of several clotting factors. Dietary deficiency or gut disease potentially causes a decrease in levels of vitamin K in the body, again affecting blood clotting.
  - *Consumption*: Clotting factors may become used up (consumed) in certain pathological situations when widespread clotting has occurred, secondary coagulopathies can then follow, causing tendency to bleed, as in DIC (see above).
  - Infectious agents: Certain viruses, such as *infectious canine hepatitis* (ICH) virus, damage blood vessel endothelial cells. This stimulates widespread clotting which uses up available clotting factors, causing secondary tendency to bleed. *Feline infectious peritonitis* (FIP) virus in cats is associated with inflammation of blood vessels (vasculitis) and this can cause diffuse clotting and thus DIC. In septicaemia, certain bacteria (such as *Salmonella* or *Leptospira*) or some bacterial toxins can similarly damage the endothelium causing widespread clotting then secondary bleeding.
  - Other severe diseases: Tissue necrosis, burns, tumours and snake venoms can initiate DIC.

- *Congenital coagulopathies*: There are a number of congenital haemophilias in animals of which *haemophilia A* and *von Wille-brand's* disease are the most common.
  - *Haemophilia A*: This is a deficiency of one of the clotting factors in the clotting cascade which is called factor VIII. The deficiency is caused by decreased synthesis or secretion, or by formation of abnormal ineffective forms of factor VIII. Haemophilia A has been recorded in dogs (mild, moderate or severe forms), cats, horses and cattle.
  - *von Willebrand's disease* (dogs): von Willebrand factor (vWF) is a glycoprotein produced by the endothelial cells and by platelet-producing megakaryocytes in bone marrow. vWf is able to bind to both platelets and endothelial cells and hence encourages platelet aggregation in the clotting process. The disease occurs in varying severity in dogs and it may even be inapparent (sub-clinical), and can be triggered by stress or other diseases.

Haemorrhage varies in significance to the animal, with some occur-rences being more harmful than others.

What factors determine the clinical significance of haemorrhage?

- *Where the bleeding occurs*: If haemorrhage is into a low-pressure area, such as the abdomen in the case of a damaged spleen or an inadequate spay ligature, then bleeding will be able to continue almost unchecked if not treated. Any clots formed may be simply 'pushed' off by the force of blood behind them. If bleeding occurs into an area which has higher local pressure, such as into a muscle in the case of bleeding around a fractured bone, for instance, a large bruise, the haemorrhage may be prevented from getting too serious because the muscle and connective tissue in the area will act like a pressure bandage, and clotting is more likely to be successful at stopping the flow.
- *How fast the bleeding occurs*: Again, this may relate to pressure in the surrounding area but also which type of vessel is bleeding. An artery will bleed faster than a vein and the blood loss will be more serious and less likely to clot successfully without treatment. As well as determining the likely success of the clotting process, the speed of blood loss will determine how sick the animal becomes as a result of the haemorrhage. An animal can adapt to slow loss of blood, such as chronic blood seepage from a small stomach ulcer. Rapid loss of blood, however, such as occurs from a ruptured spleen, is likely to cause sudden serious decrease in blood pressure, and more dramatic clinical consequences.
- *How much blood is lost*: Again, small slow losses can be compen-sated for by increased production of blood cells in the marrow and

by drinking or retaining more water. Large losses may exhaust the marrow and be more difficult for the animal to recover from without treatment.

Types of haemorrhage

Haemorrhages of different types or at different sites have specific names. As well as haemorrhage of free blood from a wound, categories of haemorrhage include:

- *Haematoma* which is localised and confined seepage of blood out of the circulation into adjacent tissues (known as *extravasation* of blood), e.g. bleeding into a muscle as a result of blunt trauma.
- *Petechiae and ecchymoses* are small haemorrhages onto or under organ surfaces. Petechiae are fine, often pinpoint haemorrhages, whilst ecchymoses are larger.
- *Melaena* is partially digested blood, which becomes black and tarry as a result of the digestive process. Melaena may be passed in the faeces of animals with stomach haemorrhage (e.g. a bleeding gastric ulcer).
- Haemorrhage into body cavities tends to be named according to the particular cavity affected, e.g. *haemothorax, haemopericardium* and *haemoperitoneum.*
- *Retinal* haemorrhages affect the back of the eye in animals with high blood pressure, and can be detected using an ophthalmoscope.

The preceding discussion has involved lack of effective clotting. If the delicate balance between clot formation and fibrinolysis shifts in favour of fibrin formation then inappropriate or excessive clotting (*thrombus formation* or *thrombosis*) may result. Thrombosis is discussed in the next section.

Thrombosis

See Box 7.13 for some important features associated with thrombosis. Note that thrombosis (formation of a thrombus) differs from blood coagulation discussed previously. Simple clots, involving activation of the coagulation cascade, can still develop outside of the circulatory system (e.g. in plain glass blood tubes or on glass slides) and can develop in animals after death. Thrombus formation, on the other hand, is specifically an abnormal process involving clotting of blood within an intact circulatory system and in a living animal.

There are certain predisposing factors, i.e. certain conditions usually need to apply, for thrombus formation. These factors are known as *Virchow's triad* (pronounced *Verr-choff*). Any one of these factors can result in thrombus formation though in many conditions more than one factor will be present.

> **Box 7.13** Key features and definitions related to thrombosis
>
> - Haemostasis = normal clotting reaction
> - Thrombosis = pathological or inappropriate clotting reaction
> - Thrombus = solid clump of blood constituents
>   - Formed within heart or vessels
>   - Formed in a living animal

Virchow's triad

For thrombi to form in the circulatory system of living animals there need to be:

- *Changes in vessel wall(s)*: Such as physical damage (trauma), chemical injury, infection or bacterial endotoxic damage, for instance.
- *Changes in flow* (slow or turbulent flow): Note that a vicious circle will be established as the resultant thrombus itself will cause turbulence.
- *Changes in blood constituents* (increased tendency to clot also called *hypercoagulability*): This happens in renal failure, diabetes mellitus, heart failure, severe trauma or burns and disseminated cancer, for instance.

A thrombus forms in layers and these can sometimes be seen under the microscope. The layers in a thrombus are due to platelets aggregating first, and then attracting fibrin with blood cells, which then attracts more platelets and so on.

Thrombi may form in the venous side of the circulation or in the arterial side. An example of venous thrombosis is *deep vein thrombosis* (DVT) when blood clots form in the veins of the legs. In humans this has been associated with protracted periods of inactivity such as recuperation after an operation or on a long haul aircraft journey. The consequences of DVT are oedema of the affected limb or pulmonary embolism (a bit of the blood clot in the leg breaks away, and passes through the heart to finally lodge in the lungs – see section *Embolism*).

Arterial thrombosis may be caused by heart disease. In this case, blood clots form on faulty heart valves due to local turbulent flow, and can break away and travel to other parts of the body in the arterial circulation. They may then lodge in vessels (*thromboembolism*, see later) and cause infarction (and ischaemia) of the affected tissue or organ.

A number of things can happen to a thrombus once it has formed (see Box 7.14), it may be broken down by phagocytic cells (like neutrophils and macrophages, see Chapter 4) completely, or partially, in this case leaving a slightly narrowed vessel. Or the thrombus may gradually be organised and become fibrous (see Chapter 6); this fibrous scar later contracting to form a permanent narrowing or blockage of the vessel. Alternatively, the thrombus may organise but become recanalised – that is little channels, lined by endothelial cells, form which allow blood to flow once more. As discussed above and in the next section, some of the thrombus may break away and lodge elsewhere (a thromboembolus).

Embolism

An embolus is *a mass of material able to lodge in a vessel and block it.* The plural of embolus is *emboli.* Emboli cause ischaemia and infarction (see earlier).

The effects of emboli depend on:

- where in the circulation they *originate* from and
- where in the circulation they *lodge*

The majority of emboli are derived from thrombi (and are known as *thromboemboli*), in other words, they are bits of larger blood clots that break away and travel in the circulation until they lodge in smaller vessels and block them.

In some heart diseases, blood clots (*thrombi*) form on the heart valves (see earlier – *arterial thrombi*). Portions of these thrombi may break away and travel in the circulation. The resulting effects depend on which side of the heart the valvular thrombi originally formed.

- Valvular thrombosis on the left side of the heart can lead to emboli in the systemic circulation.
- Valvular thrombosis on the right side of the heart can lead to emboli in the pulmonary circulation (lungs).

'Saddle thrombus' and hypertrophic cardiomyopathy in cats

An example of thromboembolic disease not uncommon in veterinary practice is so-called 'saddle' thrombus (thromboembolus in the caudal aorta or iliac arteries) in cats with the congenital heart disease *hypertrophic cardiomyopathy.* The thromboembolus interrupts blood supply to the hind legs and affected cats initially may be restless or throw themselves around (which is assumed to be due to a severe 'pins and needles' feeling in their legs). Later, if the condition progresses unchecked, there is loss of pulse in the hindlimbs, coldness of the hind paws and loss of sensation and muscle control (see Box 7.15).

As well as thrombi, other materials or substances are potential sources of emboli, which can lodge in blood vessels and block them.

Box 7.14 Fate of a thrombus

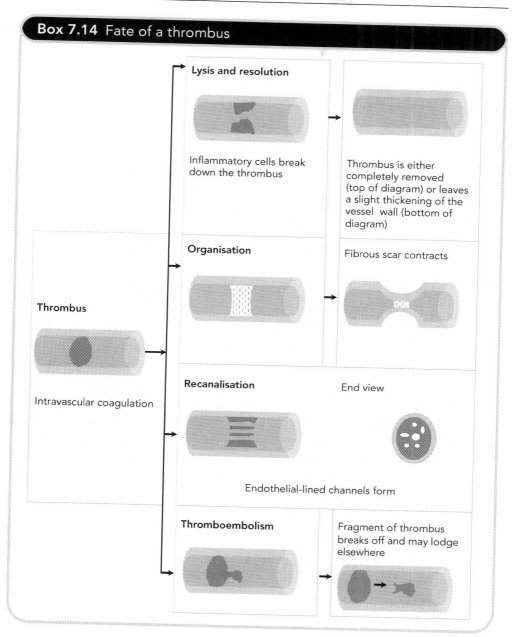

Thrombus

Intravascular coagulation

Lysis and resolution

Inflammatory cells break down the thrombus

Thrombus is either completely removed (top of diagram) or leaves a slight thickening of the vessel wall (bottom of diagram)

Organisation

Fibrous scar contracts

Recanalisation

End view

Endothelial-lined channels form

Thromboembolism

Fragment of thrombus breaks off and may lodge elsewhere

Box 7.15 'Saddle' thrombus in cats

An example of thromboembolic disease which is not uncommon in veterinary practice is the so-called 'saddle' thrombus in cats with the congenital heart disease *hypertrophic cardiomyopathy*. A thrombus forms in the heart and a thromboembolus dislodges from this primary site and enters the main artery leaving the left side of the heart – the aorta.

   The thrombus can lodge in the lower part of the caudal aorta, at the point where this artery divides to supply blood to the hind legs and tail. The unfortunate cartoon cat in the diagram below has a 'saddle' thrombus.

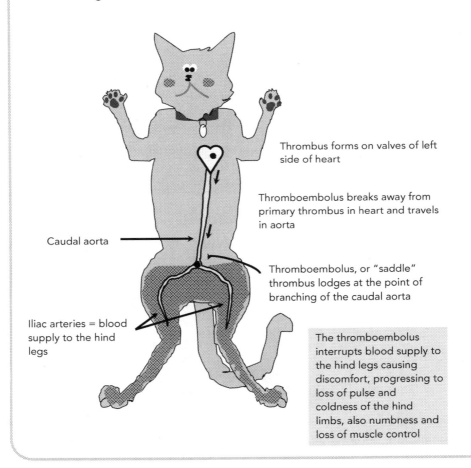

Thrombus forms on valves of left side of heart

Thromboembolus breaks away from primary thrombus in heart and travels in aorta

Caudal aorta

Thromboembolus, or "saddle" thrombus lodges at the point of branching of the caudal aorta

Iliac arteries = blood supply to the hind legs

The thromboembolus interrupts blood supply to the hind legs causing discomfort, progressing to loss of pulse and coldness of the hind limbs, also numbness and loss of muscle control

Examples of other forms of embolus

- Embolus of *tumour cells*: A malignant tumour, such as a mammary carcinoma in a dog, can invade into a blood vessel. A small embolus (metastasis) of tumour cells may then travel in the circulation to another site, commonly the lungs and establish another tumour.
- *Parasitic* emboli: In some countries where heartworm (*dirofilaria*) is common, larvae from the heartworm may travel from the heart and lodge in the capillaries of the lungs of affected dogs.
- *Fat* emboli: When a long bone fractures, fat from the central marrow cavity may enter the blood circulatory system. Fat emboli have occasionally been found in the lungs of animals injured in road traffic accidents (RTAs).
- *Infective/inflammatory* emboli: Infectious agents, necrotic tissue, leucocytes and fibrin may enter the circulation from a site of infection or inflammation; infection may be spread around the body this way (*haematogenous spread*).
- *Foreign* material: When the circulatory system is exposed by injury, injection or surgery, any foreign material could potentially enter the bloodstream and travel to another site. Some foreign matter could establish secondary granulomatous inflammation (*foreign body response* – see Chapter 4 on inflammation).
- *Fibrocartilage* emboli: when the cartilage and fibrous cushion between vertebral bones (*vertebral* or *spinal disc*) degenerates due to old age or traumatic damage in dogs, it can rupture ('slipped disc') and very occasionally small pieces of fibrocartilage enter the blood stream, and lodge somewhere else, such as the lungs.
- *Gas* emboli: This is why we are careful to expel air from syringes before giving an intravenous injection. Gas or air bubbles can lodge in the bloodstream and act as solid obstructions. This is also something that can be a problem to deep-sea divers when they come to the surface too quickly and gas bubbles expand in their blood (this condition is called 'the bends'!).

Shock

Shock is a term which is often misused. We hear about it in the newspapers or on the TV when we are told that someone who has had a traumatic or frightening experience is being 'treated for shock'. When something dramatic happens to us we are often frightened, shaky, and weak for a while afterwards and in this case the problem is perhaps more often a psychological effect – we are said to have *had* a shock.

In this chapter and in the context of the circulatory system we are referring to a different type of shock – a physiological or pathological effect. In this context *shock is defined as a state of circulatory collapse, resulting in a severe state of reduced blood perfusion of tissue blood.*

In shock, there is a mismatch between the total blood volume, and the volume of the circulatory system. In other words, the blood volume is 'too small' to fill the circulatory system, because there has been a decrease in the blood volume or because the circulatory system has effectively increased in size (by dilation of blood vessels) or because of failure of the heart to pump blood around the circulatory system. There is therefore a decreased *effective* circulating blood volume (and therefore circulation of oxygen, nutrients, warmth, waste products etc.).

There are different types of shock (Box 7.16) but many of them share similar mechanisms, so for the purposes of discussion, we can group the different forms of shock for convenience of discussion (see below). Note, however, that in some severe diseases more than one type of shock may be superimposed and keep in mind that the problem is a decreased *effective* circulating blood volume.

Hypovolaemic shock: Shock due to decreased blood volume. Hypovolaemia means decreased blood volume. Causes of hypovolaemic shock therefore include severe haemorrhage or dehydration. Hypovolaemia would also occur where there has been major leakage of fluid from the circulation into the interstitial fluid. This would occur if something caused suddenly increased permeability ('leakiness') of capillaries and this mechanism is part of the cause of shock in some fatal infections.

Vasodilation: This causes a marked increase in 'size' of the circulatory system in comparison to the amount of blood it holds; in effect, a pooling of blood in the dilated part of the circulation occurs (and therefore lack of effective circulation). In fact, it is the low-pressure capillaries that dilate. Though so small, capillaries are very numerous and have a huge potential volume, so when they are dilated they can hold a substantial amount of the animal's total blood. The blood effectively 'pools' in the capillary beds.

There are a number of examples of forms of shock where vasodilation is the mechanism.

Septic or toxic shock is caused by vasodilation of capillaries in abdominal organs. Toxins involved in toxic shock include bacterial toxins, toxins released by damaged tissue (e.g. in cases of gangrene) and some venoms. In some severe infections, toxins will cause irreversible toxic damage to vessel endothelial cells triggering DIC (see earlier discussion, this chapter, page 137). This damage will also

Box 7.16 Causes and types of shock (Part 1)

Hypovolaemic shock – shock due to decreased blood volume.

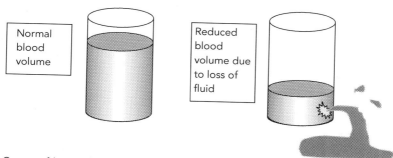

Normal blood volume

Reduced blood volume due to loss of fluid

Causes of *hypovolaemic shock* include severe haemorrhage, dehydration, marked loss of fluid from the circulation into the interstitium (e.g. due to sudden marked increase in permeability of capillaries as can occur in some fatal infections).

Shock due to vasodilation – vasodilation causes a marked increase in 'size' of the circulatory system in comparison to the amount of blood it holds. In practice, often one part of the circulatory system dilates so blood pools in the dilated part (and therefore is less available to circulate through the rest of the system).

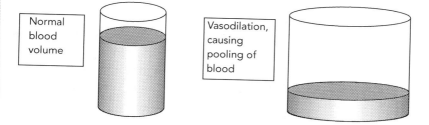

Normal blood volume

Vasodilation, causing pooling of blood

It is usually capillaries that dilate and the blood 'pools' in the capillary beds. Though so small, capillaries represent a huge potential volume because they are so numerous; when dilated, capillaries can hold a substantial amount of the animal's total blood.

Box 7.16 (*Continued*) Causes and types of shock (Part 2)

Examples of forms of shock which involve vasodilation are:

- *Septic or toxic* shock caused by vasodilation of capillaries in abdominal organs due to bacterial toxins, toxins released by damaged tissue (e.g. in cases of gangrene) and some venoms.
- *Neurogenic* shock in animals when severely frightened or traumatised, or in extreme pain. Nerves stimulate vasodilation and hence pooling of blood.
- *Anaphylactic* shock due to extreme hypersensitivity. Something to which the animal is sensitive stimulates diffuse and marked mast cell degranulation. The contents of the released mast cell granules stimulate widespread vasodilation.

  In anaphylactic shock, vasodilation may occur in the arteriolar and venous parts of the circulation as well as the capillary bed.
- *Cardiogenic shock* – acute cardiac failure causes severe marked decrease in cardiac output because the heart is suddenly unable to pump the blood effectively.

cause increased permeability of the capillaries, hence fluid loss (hypovolaemia) will compound the vasodilation.

Neurogenic shock occurs in animals when severely frightened or traumatised, or in extreme pain. Nerves stimulate vasodilation and hence pooling of blood. Neurogenic shock may compound the effects of psychological shock (fright or trauma) discussed at the start of this section.

Anaphylactic shock is an example of extreme hypersensitivity. Something to which the animal is sensitive (the allergen) stimulates marked mast cell degranulation (see Chapter 4, Inflammation, for actions of mast cell granules). The contents of the released mast cell granules stimulate vasodilation. In anaphylactic shock, vasodilation may occur in the arteriolar and venous parts of the circulation as well.

Cardiogenic shock – acute cardiac failure causes severe marked decrease in cardiac output because the heart is suddenly unable to pump the blood effectively.

Pathological effects of shock

Many of the pathological effects of shock result from the decreased *effective* transport functions of the circulatory system (see again the functions of the circulatory system at the start of this chapter). So, in a severely shocked animal the following pathological effects may result:

- Ischaemia due to decreased O_2 supply causes necrosis, especially in the most vulnerable organs (brain and heart).

- Decreased oxidative metabolism (and increased anaerobic metabolism) which causes altered acid–base levels in the blood. The pH of the blood decreases and becomes dangerously acid (*acidosis*) which is harmful to a number of cell functions. The acid–base levels cannot be corrected as they normally would by the kidney, gut and lungs, as the function of these organs is also compromised by decreased blood perfusion. Altered oxidative metabolism also causes *hypoglycaemia* (low blood sugar levels).
- The sympathetic (autonomic) nervous system and hormones divert blood from non-essential areas such as muscle and skin to vital organs such as the brain.
- The sympathetic nervous system may also cause an increase in the heart rate and the respiratory rate to try to compensate for the reduced circulation.
- In the later stages, *hypoxia* (O_2 depletion) causes irreversible paralysis of the peripheral circulation (*flaccid vasodilation*) which causes stagnation of blood in capillaries (*sludging*).

The clinical signs of shock

The signs are similar in man or animals and if you have completed first aid training you will be familiar with them.

Note that in some cases clinical signs are specific to a particular cause of shock (e.g. hypovolaemic, toxic, infectious, cardiogenic or anaphylactic shocks) but the general effects on the circulation are similar in most if not all cases:

- cold extremities
- core temperature high or low depending on cause of shock
- shivering in early stages
- heart rate may be increased or may be irregular and/or decreased
- weak peripheral pulse
- collapsed circulation (it may be hard to find a vein for intravenous injections or infusions)
- respiratory rate may be increased initially but may decrease if animal loses consciousness
- pale or discoloured (brick red or even blue) mucous membranes
- slow capillary refill times
- lethargy, lack of interest in surroundings, depression (and these effects may be accompanied or exacerbated by signs of pain, if shock is due to blood loss after trauma)
- loss of consciousness
- muscle weakness
- decreased urine production
- decreased blood pressure

You may be able to add further signs you have or will see in relation to shock resulting from particular causes.

Summary of key points in Chapter 7

- Oedema is accumulation of excessive interstitial fluid to cause a soft pitting swelling of affected areas. There are different causes of oedema but in all, the lymphatic circulation is unable to adequately remove excess fluid from the tissues.
- Ischaemia is decreased blood flow (*perfusion*) and resulting decreased supply of vital nutrients, especially oxygen, to the area. Infarction is death (necrosis) of the area as a result of ischaemia. A period of ischaemia may not cause infarction if it is of short duration or in a tissue with a low metabolic rate.
- Coagulopathies are disorders of the clotting (coagulation) mechanism resulting from deficiency or infectiveness of any stage of the clotting process. Coagulopathies are *acquired* or *congenital*.
- Haemorrhage may result from coagulopathy or from trauma, ulceration or rupture of a neoplasm.
- Thrombosis is a pathological clotting reaction resulting in the formation of a thrombus within the heart or blood vessels of a living animal. Changes in the vessel wall, the blood flow, or in the constituency of the blood promote thrombosis.
- An embolus is a mass of material able to lodge in a vessel and block it. Emboli cause ischaemia and infarction. Most emboli are derived from thrombi (thromboemboli). Examples of other forms of embolus are tumour cells, parasite larvae, fat emboli, infective or inflammatory material, foreign material and gas.
- Shock is a state of circulatory collapse resulting in severely reduced perfusion of tissue. In shock, there is a mismatch between the total blood volume and the volume of the circulatory system. There are a number of causes of shock though the effects and clinical signs are similar in each.

Test yourself questions on Chapter 7

1. Answer the following true/false questions.
   i. Capillaries represent a very large total volume of the blood circulatory system.
   ii. Capillary beds carry blood from the venous circulation to the arterial circulation.
   iii. Capillary walls are composed of layers of smooth muscle, fibrous tissue and basement membranes.
   iv. Capillary walls are normally impermeable to fluid.
   v. Lymph vessels have thicker walls than blood vessels because they are under higher hydrostatic pressure.
   vi. The lymph system communicates with the blood circulatory system, and thus lymph fluid drains into the blood stream.
   vii. Lymph vessels have lymph nodes at intervals, which act as filters and are important in the function of the immune system.
   viii. Oedema is the accumulation of interstitial fluid in the tissues which causes a soft swelling of the tissue, which can be 'pitted'.
   ix. In non-inflammatory oedema in which the endothelial lining of the capillaries remains intact the resultant oedema fluid tends to be low in protein and usually does not contain cells.
   x. Oedema is always life-threatening.

2. a. In relation to decreased blood supply to the tissues, contrast the terms *ischaemia* and *infarction*.
   b. List six common causes of ischaemia.
   c. What is meant by a global infarction?
   d. Draw a very simple flow diagram to illustrate the stages of development of an infarct.

3. a. What part does the soluble protein, fibrinogen, play in blood coagulation?
   b. Briefly indicate why vitamin K is important to blood coagulation.

4. a. Discuss the factors which determine the clinical significance of haemorrhage in animals.
   b. A dog in your care develops black tarry faeces – what would you suspect was happening in the digestive tract, and in which part of the tract would you suspect it was occurring? How would your answer differ if there was fresh blood in the faeces?

Test yourself questions on Chapter 7 (Continued)

5. a. What is meant by embolus?
    b. Briefly describe formation of a thromboembolus in the case of heart valve disorders.
    c. Give three examples of other forms of embolus.
6. a. Define 'shock'.
    b. Briefly outline the various main types of shock according to the way they develop.
    c. Give five typical clinical signs of shock.

Chapter 8
Disorders of Cell/Tissue Growth

<u>Atrophy, hypertrophy, hyperplasia and metaplasia</u>

<u>Neoplasia</u>

Neoplasia terminology
Stages of tumour development
Loss of control of cell proliferation
Loss of normal cell differentiation
What causes gene damage and allows a tumour to develop?
Modifiers of tumour growth
Rates of tumour growth
Tumour growth patterns
Metastasis
Routes of metastasis
Diagnosis of neoplasms in veterinary general practice

> ### Aims of Chapter 8
>
> - To introduce the concepts of reversible and irreversible changes in cell or tissue growth or size as responses to stimuli
> - To define some of the most commonly encountered changes in cell or tissue growth or size – atrophy, hypertrophy, hyperplasia, metaplasia and neoplasia
> - To discuss causes, development and effects of these changes and to become familiar with common examples

In Chapter 3, we discussed changes in cells in response to stimuli and noted that these changes may be reversible or non-reversible. Reversible changes are non-permanent changes from which the cell may recover or revert to normal once the stimulus stops. In some cases reversible changes include *adaptations* of the cell to a new environment, in which case the stimulus is the change in the environment. These changes help the cell to survive and cope with an altered environment. If the change in the environment continues, the cell will not actually revert to its previous normal state but will adapt to the new requirements placed upon it and establish a new 'normal' in terms of function and metabolism. So, in summary, cellular adaptation means reversible changes in cells in response to a physiological or injurious stimulus.

Reversible cell adaptations include degenerations (discussed in Chapter 3) and changes in growth or size, and these are discussed in the next section.

Atrophy, hypertrophy, hyperplasia and metaplasia

Atrophy, hypertrophy, hyperplasia and metaplasia are all adaptive changes in cells which help the cell to cope with an alteration in its environment. We will discuss each in turn, starting with a definition of each term (see also Box 8.1).

Atrophy is *shrinkage* in the size of cells (and therefore the tissue of which the cell forms part) in response to a stimulus. There are a number of causes of atrophy; these and some examples are shown in Box 8.2. Note that many of these causes of atrophy are interrelated, e.g. pressure on an area, such as a limb with a tight bandage, involves reduced blood and nerve supply but also muscle atrophy due to the animal not being able to use and exercise the limb normally.

Box 8.1 Atrophy, hypertrophy, hyperplasia and metaplasia

Atrophy, hypertrophy, hyperplasia and metaplasia are adaptive changes in cells which help the cell to cope with an alteration in its environment.

Atrophy = *shrinkage* in the *size* of cells (and therefore the tissue of which the cell forms part) in response to a stimulus.
   There are a number of causes of atrophy such as disuse, loss of blood or nerve supply, inadequate nutrition, decreased hormone supply, aging and pressure.

Atrophy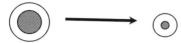

Hypertrophy = *increase in size* of cells in response to a stimulus.
   Hypertrophy may be normal (*physiological*), e.g. muscle development with exercise or changes in the uterus in pregnancy.
   Hypertrophy may also be considered abnormal (*pathological*), e.g. heart muscle in cats with hypertrophic cardiomyopathy.
   Hypertrophy may occur most in *stable* cell populations, that is cells that do not undergo division (*mitosis*) readily.

Hypertrophy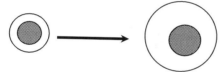

Hyperplasia = *increase in the number* of cells, e.g. in lactating mammary glands, in bone marrow (production of more red blood cells) in long-standing anaemia, in the liver after toxic damage, or hyperplasia of the gums in chronic gum and dental disease.
   Hyperplasia tends to occur most in *labile* cell populations, which are able to divide readily by mitosis.
   Sometimes, hypertrophy and hyperplasia will occur together.

Hyperplasia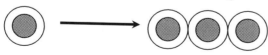

Metaplasia = *conversion of one mature tissue type into a different type*, such as alteration of an epithelium (e.g. the lining of the urinary bladder) to a tougher more protective (squamous) one in response to, for instance, chronic inflammation (presence of bladder stones).

Metaplasia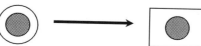

Box 8.2 Causes of atrophy

Disuse	May happen in the muscles of a limb encased in a plaster cast
Loss of nerve supply	May affect muscles in a limb when the main nerve plexus has been damaged in a RTA
Decreased blood supply	If the blood supply to an area is impaired by a vessel blockage then atrophy of the affected part may ensue (note that if the blood supply is completely cut off ischaemia and infarction are possible – see Chapter 6)
Inadequate nutrition	This relates to inadequate blood supply. An example of this is atrophy of the liver in a puppy with a portosystemic shunt. The shunt diverts blood away from the liver so that the liver cells are deprived of nutrition
Decreased hormone stimulation	For instance, mammary glands of bitches tend to atrophy once they have been spayed
Aging	Muscles tend to atrophy with age
Pressure	The atrophying effect of pressure may relate to effects of impaired blood supply, nerve supply or disuse (see above)

Hypertrophy is the *increase in size* of cells in response to a stimulus. Hypertrophy may be normal (physiological), such as muscle development with exercise or development of the mucosal lining of the uterus with pregnancy. Hypertrophy may also be considered abnormal (pathological), such as in heart muscle in a condition in cats called hypertrophic cardiomyopathy. The heart muscle becomes hypertrophied, possibly as an inherited condition, and the heart gradually fails. (See also discussion of 'saddle' thrombus in Chapter 7.)

Hypertrophy may occur most in stable cell populations (see Chapter 6), that is ones which undergo division (mitosis) slightly less readily.

Hyperplasia, on the other hand, is *increase in the number* of cells. The mammary gland undergoes hyperplasia during lactation as a normal physiological part of the reproductive cycle. Other tissues will respond to pathological stimuli by hyperplasia, such as bone marrow producing more red blood cells in chronic anaemia or the liver regenerating to replace cells damaged by toxins. In some cases, the response may be excessive, such as hyperplasia of the gums in chronic dental disease. This causes firm nodules of gum tissue to form around the teeth, which entrap more food and bacteria and can exacerbate the inflammation. Hyperplasia tends to occur most in labile cell populations, able to divide readily by mitosis, though note that in some cell types and under some conditions hypertrophy and hyperplasia will occur together.

As noted above, the liver readily undergoes hyperplasia, though a particular example of somewhat marked hyperplasia in the liver is the condition of nodular liver regeneration, already discussed in Chapter 6.

Metaplasia is conversion of one mature tissue type into another different type, such as alteration of an epithelium, for example the lining of the urinary bladder, to a tougher more protective (squamous) one in response to, for instance, chronic inflammation due to presence of bladder stones.

Now, we move on to a very important non-reversible change in cell growth and number, that of neoplasia (cancer or tumour formation).

Neoplasia

Neoplasia is the proliferation of *abnormal* cells to form *neoplasms* (cancers or tumours) (Box 8.3). Unlike the reversible changes, atrophy, hypertrophy, hyperplasia and metaplasia, discussed earlier in this chapter, neoplasia is a non-reversible change and neoplastic cells cannot revert to normal once the stimulus is removed. In fact, neoplastic changes (*transformations*) are genetic mutations and become part of the genetic make-up of the neoplastic cells, and as such are passed on to new cells when the neoplastic cell divides. What this means is that a tumour originates from one cell which *transformed* to a neoplastic type and continued dividing to produce clones of itself.

Normal cells communicate with each other and tend to grow in a coordinated manner, stopping division when no more cells are required, but neoplastic cells lack this coordination with normal tissue and go on growing and dividing in an uncontrolled manner, often to the detriment of the normal tissues surrounding them, as we shall see later.

Neoplasia terminology

Let us start this discussion of neoplasia by clarifying some terminology. First of all, what is the difference between tumours, cancers and neoplasms? Well, *neoplasm* is the term used to describe a mass of cells which are growing as a result of a neoplastic transformation. Neoplasms may be malignant or benign.

Cancer is a less formal but highly familiar term. It tends to be used to denote malignant neoplasms and is a term that is often quite frightening for owners. *Tumour* is again a highly familiar and historic term but

Box 8.3 Neoplasia

Neoplasia = uncontrolled proliferation of *abnormal* cells to form *neoplasms*.

Neoplasia is a non-reversible change; the neoplastic cells cannot revert to normal once the stimulus to divide is removed.

Neoplastic cells have genetic mutations (*transformations*) which can be passed on to new cells when the neoplastic cell divides.

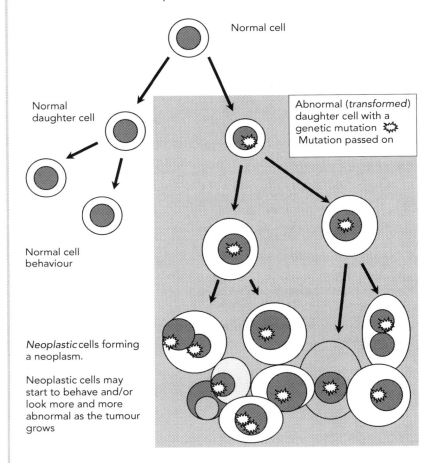

Normal cell

Normal daughter cell

Abnormal (*transformed*) daughter cell with a genetic mutation
Mutation passed on

Normal cell behaviour

Neoplastic cells forming a neoplasm.

Neoplastic cells may start to behave and/or look more and more abnormal as the tumour grows

Thus, tumours originate from one transformed cell which continued to divide and produce clones of itself.

Normal cells communicate with each other and grow in an orderly and coordinated manner; neoplastic cells lack this coordination and continue to divide in an uncontrolled manner, often to the detriment of adjacent normal tissues.

it is in actual fact usually mis-used. Tumour is really a non-specific term meaning a 'swelling' in the body. It could mean a neoplasm (benign or malignant), but strictly speaking it could equally mean an abscess, a swollen lymph node, or a focal fluid accumulation – anything that causes a firm local swelling.

Recall that one of the cardinal signs of inflammation (see Chapter 4) is 'swelling', referring to the accumulation of inflammatory exudate, and that this phenomenon is also referred to in some older texts by the classical term *tumor*.

Although not strictly speaking correct, tumour is commonly used in the context of neoplasia, and certainly most owners will be familiar with this meaning and are often slightly more comfortable with the use of this word. Both these familiar terms will be used during the rest of this chapter, but in all cases we are referring to neoplastic growth.

Tumour nomenclature

Tumours are named according to the neoplastic cell of which they are made up; in other words, the cell which *transformed* and divided to produce the tumour. The name is modified according to the broad category of cell type to which the neoplastic cell belongs – *epithelial* or *mesenchymal* (see Box 8.4 for definitions of these terms). The name is further modified according to whether the tumour is benign or malignant. The terms in italics in Box 8.4 are used at the end of the tumour name and you can see that they convey quite a bit of information about the tumour.

Box 8.4 Tumour nomenclature

| Cell | Tumour | |
	Benign	Malignant
Epithelial*	-oma	-(adeno)carcinoma*
Mesenchymal¶	-oma	- sarcoma

* Epithelial cells are 'covering' cells, such as the cells of the epidermis of the skin, the respiratory epithelium which lines the trachea (windpipe) or the intestinal epithelium.

All glands in the body are also lined by epithelial cells and these can, in certain circumstances, transform and form neoplasms. Inserting the term 'adeno' into the tumour name indicates that it is formed from a *glandular* epithelium.

¶ Whereas epithelial cells are covering cells, mesenchymal cells are structural or 'filling in' cells. Mesenchymal cells include bone, cartilage, collagenous fibrous tissue, but also the red and white blood cells and the cells from which they develop (bone marrow or haematopoietic cells).

The broad terms *epithelial* and *mesenchymal* used in Box 8.4 stem from terminology used in *embryology*, the study of the development of embryos.

This business of naming tumours might all seem a bit confusing, so consider some examples; you may already have come across some of these tumours during your clinical work. Refer to the text box above and try to follow the terminology used to name these tumours.

Examples of naming of tumours

Osteosarcoma – 'osteo' means concerning the bones, so the transformed cell was a bone cell; 'sarcoma' means a malignant mesenchymal cell tumour.

Sebaceous adenoma – a benign glandular epithelial cell tumour, specifically the transformed cell was a cell of the sebaceous glands in the skin.

Mammary adenocarcinoma – a malignant epithelial cell tumour formed from a transformed mammary gland cell.

Dermal fibroma – a benign tumour of fibrous tissue of the skin's dermis; the transformed cell was of the type involved in producing collagen in fibrous tissue.

Note that the process of tumour development is known as *carcinogenesis* and something that acts as a trigger for a neoplasm to develop is described as being *carcinogenic* – this refers to its potential to cause any type of neoplasm, and not just carcinomas as the term suggests.

Note also that pathologists sometimes use names that seem to be exceptions to this terminology and could imply a malignant tumour is benign – in these cases we usually clarify what type of tumour we mean, such as '*malignant* melanoma'. Though lymphoma remains an accepted exception!

Do not get too alarmed if this naming seems confusing at this stage, you will become familiar with these terms during your clinical work.

There are recognised stages in tumour development and these are discussed in the next section.

Stages of tumour development

Study of tumour development in men and animals is an important and growing area of research and has led to advances in cancer management, more sophisticated treatments and, for many tumours, a better prognosis than previously. In this section, we discuss some of what is currently known about development of tumours.

Tumour development occurs in stages (Box 8.5), requiring first of all an *initiating* event (examples are discussed below), which leads to

---

Box 8.5 Summary of the stages of tumour development

Initiation	A trigger factor or event that causes irreversible *genetic changes* producing a transformed cell
Promotion	A factor or event that causes the transformed cell to *proliferate*, forming a neoplasm
Progression	Spontaneous occurrence of *new genetic mutations* in offspring of the original transformed cell, possibly increasing malignant behaviour of the tumour

damage to the DNA in the genes of a single cell in a population. This *initiated* (or transformed) cell looks and, initially after transformation at least, behaves normally, harbouring its abnormal genetic material for some time, maybe even years, without ill-effect to the animal.

This genetic abnormality gives the cell an advantage over its normal neighbours so that at some stage, it will start to proliferate in response to another stimulus. This stage is called *promotion*. Promotion is an event that causes the transformed cell to proliferate producing a neoplasm, and in so doing passing its genetic abnormalities on to its offspring.

Later still, there is likely to be a stage called *progression* which is formation of new genetic mutations, the most 'successful' of which (in neoplasia terms), will encourage proliferation of increasingly aberrant cell types leading to increasing 'aggressiveness' or malignancy in the tumour.

We will look at what can cause gene damage (the initiators and promoters of tumour development) in the next section, but first let us just consider in what ways tumour cells differ from normal.

Two fundamental alterations to normal cell behaviour underlie tumour development. Neoplasia involves:

- loss of control of cell proliferation and
- loss of normal cell differentiation

Loss of control of cell proliferation

Neoplastic cells do not grow and divide according to the body's requirements as other cell types do, they can continue dividing and growing without regard for the control processes that act on normal tissues.

Box 8.6 illustrates the stages that a normal cell must undergo when it divides into two new daughter cells; this process is known as the *cell cycle*.

Box 8.6 The cell cycle and loss of its control in neoplasia

Many cells are able to divide and therefore reproduce themselves (see also Chapter 6). Cells that are not involved in producing eggs or sperm in the reproductive organs, in other words, most cells of the rest of the body (known as somatic cells) divide by mitosis. Mitosis is a complex process involving the cell dividing into two equal parts. This might sound simple, but think what might be involved in this process and what the result would be if the process did not go smoothly or correctly! The nuclear material (DNA) of the cell must be duplicated carefully and then shared out equally so that each daughter cell gets all of the information and components it needs to function properly. The cytoplasm and the cell membrane also need to be divided up.

The division process occurs in a carefully organised sequence of events which occur as part of the *cell cycle*, see diagram and the explanation of each significant stage below.

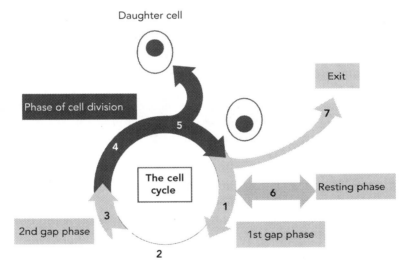

Phase of production of DNA

At point **1** in the diagram above, a cell is 'instructed' by various chemical messengers (growth factors) to start the process of division and to proceed through a temporary 'gap' phase to the second phase – that of production of DNA (**2**). There then follows another gap phase (**3**) and then the cell enters the phase of division (**4**), in which the nucleus and cytoplasm are split, culminating in two new daughter cells (**5**). Each of these new cells can then proceed through the cell cycle. Alternatively, cells can take a break from the cell cycle at this point and enter a resting phase (**6**). This resting phase is of variable length and accounts for the differing readiness to divide of *labile* and *stable* cell populations in the body (see Chapter 6). Growth factors wake a cell out of its resting phase and stimulate it to start the phase of DNA production.

Box 8.6 *(Continued)* The cell cycle and loss of its control in neoplasia

Certain cells may leave the cell cycle permanently (**7**) by entering the ominously named phase of *terminal differentiation*. Terminally differentiated cells cannot re-enter the cell cycle once they have opted to leave it. These cells forfeit the ability to divide and die off at the end of their lifespans (permanent cells are of this type, Chapter 6).

Control of the cell cycle

The cell cycle is somewhat of a series of challenges for the cell and only cells which successfully pass all the tests manage to complete the cycle, ending up as two cells!
    So how is this controlled?
    As already indicated, cells are stimulated to start the process of division by growth factors acting at **1** (and **6**) on our simplified diagram of the cell cycle.
    But as well as stimulatory factors, there are also checkpoints along the way which monitor the cell's progress and allow it to continue to the next stage or slow it down (or even stop it going any further).
    These factors can be summed up as *growth-promoting factors* and *growth-inhibiting factors*, and cell proliferation depends on a **balance** between the activity of these two types of factors – summarised in the following cartoon.

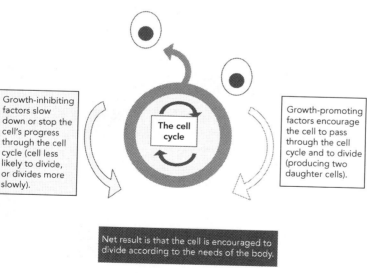

Growth-inhibiting factors slow down or stop the cell's progress through the cell cycle (cell less likely to divide, or divides more slowly).

The cell cycle

Growth-promoting factors encourage the cell to pass through the cell cycle and to divide (producing two daughter cells).

Net result is that the cell is encouraged to divide according to the needs of the body.

Growth-promoting factors encourage the cell to keep moving through the cell cycle. Conversely, if they detect a fault in a cell's DNA during the cell cycle, *growth-inhibiting factors* will slow down its progress allowing time for repair of the fault. If the fault cannot be rectified, these factors can stop the process and can even direct the cell to kill itself to avoid the fault being passed on. Growth inhibiting factors thus provide a sort of quality control system for dividing cells.

Box 8.6 (*Continued*) The cell cycle and loss of its control in neoplasia

Neoplastic cells proliferate in an unregulated fashion and not according to the body's requirements as other cell types do. This is because transformed (neoplastic) cells tend to have *abnormal* (mutated) growth-promoting and growth-inhibiting genes so that uncontrolled division of the cells is possible, thus leading to development of a tumour. What can happen is that a neoplastic cell loses growth-inhibiting genes, or its growth-promoting genes become more active, thus pushing the cell through the cell cycle more often and at a faster rate (and in an uncontrolled manner).

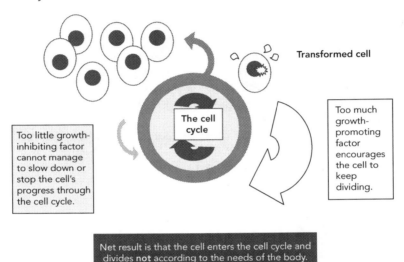

Transformed cell

The cell cycle

Too little growth-inhibiting factor cannot manage to slow down or stop the cell's progress through the cell cycle.

Too much growth-promoting factor encourages the cell to keep dividing.

Net result is that the cell enters the cell cycle and divides **not** according to the needs of the body.

Even in a normal animal a small amount of genetic damage occurs as time goes by and the animal ages, but as we discussed above, there are checkpoints in the cell cycle which monitor the 'health' of the DNA and many harmful abnormalities can be detected and the damage repaired or the cell directed to destroy itself.

Because transformed cells are dividing without adequate regulation and often more rapidly than normal cells, they are even more prone to make mistakes in dividing up their DNA, and thus even more marked genetic abnormalities can occur. Thus more and more genetic mutations develop during the *progression* stage of tumour development.

Control of cell proliferation normally depends on a balance between certain genetically determined growth-promoting factors and growth-inhibiting factors. These factors act at various stages on the cell cycle of the dividing cells to encourage them to continue with the cycle and divide, or to stop the process and remain undivided, according to the body's needs.

Transformed cells which go on to start neoplasms have abnormal growth-promoting genes and growth-inhibiting genes, so that uncontrolled and often rapid division of the cells is possible.

Even in a normal animal a small amount of genetic damage will occur as the animal ages. There are checkpoints in the cell cycle which monitor the 'health' of the DNA and harmful abnormalities can often be detected and the damage repaired. If it cannot be repaired then the cell selflessly destroys itself.

Because transformed cells are dividing in an unregulated way, they are *even more* prone to make mistakes, and *even more* marked genetic abnormalities can develop. As stated above, such abnormal cells would normally be destroyed by various checks in the normal cell proliferation system, but in neoplasia the abnormal cells 'slip through the net' and are allowed to survive. This is how more and more genetic mutations develop during the progression stage of tumour development.

Loss of normal cell differentiation

Consider one of the fertilised eggs or ova in a bitch's uterus after a successful mating. That single cell contains all the genetic information required to make a whole dog, half from the mother (from the unfertilised egg) and half from the father (from the sperm). The egg develops into an embryo by dividing and producing more and more cells, but not all of these cells will look the same or be performing the same functions in the developing embryo and later in the fully formed dog. Some of these cells will have the ability to secrete hormones, some will line the gut and will be absorptive, some will become muscle cells and be able to contract, and some will transmit nerve impulses and so on. The cells are said to *differentiate*, in other words, to follow a particular 'career' path. All these cells have the same genetic information hidden away inside them; each cell *could* potentially make a whole dog, but as lots of cells actually work together to make the dog, each cell only needs to use a small percentage of their genetic information according to the requirements of their location and functions.

Neoplastic cells, on the other hand, show abnormal differentiation such as inappropriate proliferation, abnormal growth patterns or inappropriate hormone production. The reason they do this is because they re-awaken some of their 'dormant' genetic material; genetic information that a normal cell at that site and doing that job would not need to utilise. The cells become 'less well differentiated', and in terms of the tumour they form, the poorer the cellular differentiation, the poorer the prognosis for the animal, because the more inappropriately behaved the cells are going to be. We will discuss this aspect of tumours a little later in this chapter (see 'What effects do tumours have on animals?'and 'paraneoplastic effects').

What causes gene damage and allows a tumour to develop?

A number of agents or risk factors have been associated with tumour development, and the list may grow as research identifies more potential carcinogens. A few carcinogens are listed below, but note that more than one step is required in development of tumours and some agents will act as initiators and some as promoters.

Examples of potential carcinogens
- *Chemicals*: For example, chemical factors contained in bracken, which can cause bladder cancer in cattle which graze on the fern. Also, the chemicals in tobacco smoke are potent carcinogens for humans.
- *Viruses*: Examples include Papillomavirus (the 'wart' virus, related to the virus that causes human cervical cancer) and retroviruses (feline leukaemia virus, FeLV).
- *Radiation*: Isotopes and ultraviolet light (sunlight).
- *Hormones*: For instance steroid hormone and growth hormone – both these types of hormone may be implicated in mammary tumours in some species.
- *Bacteria and parasites*: A species of bacterium called *Helicobacter* may be involved in stomach cancer in some species. In warm climates, infection of dogs by a nematode (roundworm) causes large granulomas (see *chronic inflammation*, Chapter 4) to form in the oesophagus. Occasionally, infection also causes oesophageal sarcomas to develop.

Modifiers of tumour growth

- Most tumours are more likely to occur with increasing age of animal. This effect may be due to accumulation of genetic damage with time, decreased immune function, or to a delay between initiation (transformation) and promotion and clinically detectable tumour. Although there are certain tumours which affect only young animals, e.g. some brain tumours in young dogs, histiocytoma in the skin of dogs and certain lymphoid tumours in cats.
- There are breed predispositions for some tumours, such as osteosarcoma in large breeds of dog, brain tumours in some brachycephalic breeds, and a tumour called malignant histiosarcoma in Bernese Mountain dogs. With the development of the canine genome project, the genetic basis of these breed-specific tumours may well become known.

Rates of tumour growth

You may already be aware that tumours tend to grow at different rates. Often the most harmful ones grow more rapidly. Less harmful tumours are often slow growing or remain almost unchanged for long periods of time.

The rate at which a tumour grows depends to a large extent on the rate of tumour cell proliferation, in other words, the speed with which cells divide and form new cells which are also capable of division. There are, however, factors which can modify this rate of proliferation. Because they are dividing in an uncontrolled and uncoordinated manner, when tumour cells divide they are not necessarily dividing effectively. This means that the offspring of tumour cell division may not inherit all the genetic material they require for full function. Not all tumour cells, for instance, have the ability to divide successfully and some cells may be so defective that they cannot survive, and will die anyway.

Another reason for the difference in rate of tumour growth relates to differences in the adequacy of the blood supply of the tumour. Tumour cells, like all cells in the body, require a blood supply to provide nutrients and oxygen and to remove waste products of metabolism (see *angiogenesis* below). Fast-growing tumours are said to 'outgrow' their own blood supply. Blood vessels in tumours tend to be rather irregular and easily compressed and can be occluded by the pressure of rapidly proliferating tumour cells. This means that larger or more rapidly growing tumours may contain areas of necrosis (infarction – see Chapter 7) due to ischaemia.

Angiogenesis

'angio' concerned with the blood vessels; '-genesis' to produce or bring forth.

As previously pointed out in the discussion of rates of tumour growth above, tumour cells require a blood supply to provide nutrients and oxygen and to remove waste products of metabolism just as do normal cells of the body. Tumour cells secrete a chemical messenger which encourages new blood vessels to sprout from venules and capillaries in adjacent tissue (see Box 8.7). This process is known as *angiogenesis* and the factor the cells secrete is called, appropriately, *tumour angiogenesis factor (TAF)*.

Without a blood supply, tumours would not be able to expand beyond a few millimetres diameter, needing to rely on diffusion of gases from the interstitial fluid. A blood supply is also required by the tumours for sustained tumour growth and for tumour spread (metastasis),

Box 8.7 Tumours stimulate their own blood supply (angiogenesis)

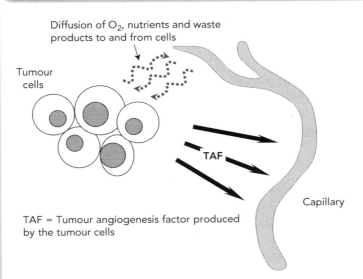

Diffusion of O_2, nutrients and waste products to and from cells

Tumour cells

TAF

Capillary

TAF = Tumour angiogenesis factor produced by the tumour cells

In the diagram above, a small cluster of tumour cells are secreting tumour angiogenesis factor (TAF).

Below, the TAF has stimulated a small vessel to sprout from the adjacent capillary. This small vessel is growing into the developing tumour, supplying the oxygen and nutrients, and removing waste from the tumour cells. This allows the tumour to grow in size from just a few clustered cells as shown above.

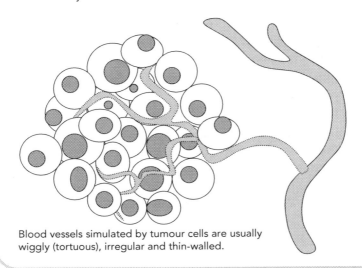

Blood vessels simulated by tumour cells are usually wiggly (tortuous), irregular and thin-walled.

though note that angiogenesis occurs in both benign and malignant tumours.

You are probably aware of specific tumours of blood vessels (hae-mangioma and haemangiosarcoma). In these tumours the neoplastic cells are transformed blood vessel cells. In angiogenesis the cells form-ing the blood vessels are not neoplastic, they are simply responding to instructions issued by the neoplastic cells.

The blood vessels formed are sometimes not very efficient. They may be small and tortuous (wiggly) and often leaky, as though the cells forming them do not receive very clear instructions from the tumour cells. This is partly why rapidly growing tumours may develop central areas of ischaemic necrosis.

Tumour growth patterns

Tumours have a number of different growth patterns (see Box 8.8). These growth patterns are usually related to whether the tumour is benign or malignant, though growth patterns may also be dictated by location. Within tissue, benign tumours tend to form discrete masses, with well-defined margins. So, for instance, a benign mammary tumour may be palpated as a firm round structure, which is freely movable un-der the skin. They tend to enlarge by expanding and sometimes com-pressing normal tissues around them, often forming a fibrous capsule, but in any case there is usually a distinct border between tumour and normal tissue. At surgery, such a benign mass is easy to remove and is often said to 'shell out' easily. On organ surfaces, benign tumours are often well-defined *domes* or *plaques*, though some protrude (some-times markedly) from the surface and may be described as *peduncu-lated*. If they have a 'frilly' surface, somewhat like a sea anemone, they may be described as *papillary*.

Malignant tumours, on the other hand, are usually less discrete. Within tissues they often extend in an irregular manner into adjacent normal tissue; this is known as local invasion. It can be harder to see or feel the edge of such invasive tumours and because of this it can be harder to completely excise them at surgery. The surgeon will need to take a wide margin of apparently normal tissue to try to ensure com-plete removal of the tumour. On tissue surfaces, malignant tumours are more likely to be ulcerated or eroded and to get secondarily in-fected. Note that there can be exceptions to these general rules, so be careful about giving owners advice as to whether the tumour is likely to be benign or malignant until you are sure.

Metastasis

As discussed in the last sections, some non-benign tumours will invade locally by sending tendrils of tumour cells into adjacent normal tissue.

Box 8.8 Tumour growth patterns

The growth pattern (shape) of a tumour often relates to whether the tumour is benign or malignant (though location may also affect the way a tumour grows).

Benign tumours tend to grow as well-defined and discrete masses that may be freely movable under the skin or in other loose tissues, or that can be readily dissected out at surgery – i.e. they 'shell-out' easily.

These tumours tend to enlarge by expansion, sometimes compressing adjacent normal tissues, and often having a fibrous capsule around them. The capsule forms where the tumour has compressed normal tissues so much that the cells die (*necrosis* due to pressure, see Chapter 3) and fibrosis occurs (see Chapter 6).

It is usually easy to recognise where tumour ends and normal tissue begins!

(a) A small benign tumour (grey 'cells') growing amongst normal (white) cells of a tissue. Benign tumours tend to grow by expansion (shown by arrows).

(b) The same benign tumour shown in **(a)** has now grown a bit bigger and has compressed the normal cells around it.

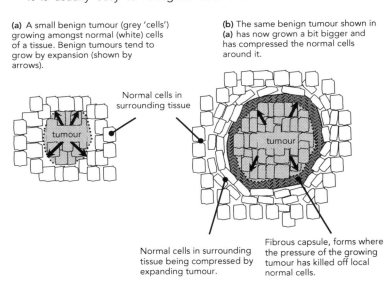

Normal cells in surrounding tissue

tumour

tumour

Normal cells in surrounding tissue being compressed by expanding tumour.

Fibrous capsule, forms where the pressure of the growing tumour has killed off local normal cells.

On the surface of organs, benign tumours may grow as simple *domes* or *plaques*.

Occasionally, they may protrude from the surface and are then described as *pedunculated*. If they have a rough or 'frilly' surface they may be described as *papillary*.

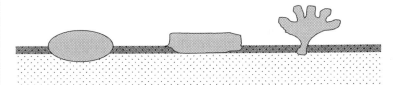

(c) A small benign tumour growing as a dome-shaped structure on the surface of a tissue or organ, e.g. the skin.

(d) A small benign tumour growing as a flattened plaque on the surface of a tissue or organ.

(e) A small benign tumour growing as a pedunculated structure on the surface of a tissue or organ.

All of these tumours have well-defined deep edges, and a capsule may form at the deep edges of the tumours as they compress normal cells (as in **(b)** above).
Once again, these tumours should be relatively easy to dissect out at surgery.

Box 8.8 (Continued) Tumour growth patterns

Malignant tumours are usually less well-defined, and often extend in an irregular manner into adjacent normal tissue – this is known as *local invasion*. It can be harder to see or feel the edge of tumours that grow by invasion and because of this they can also be more difficult to dissect out completely at surgery. The surgeon will usually try to remove a wide margin of apparently normal tissue to try to make sure that the tumour has been adequately removed.

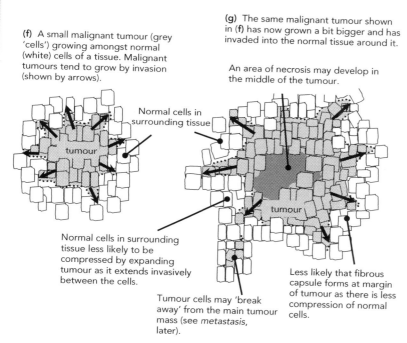

(f) A small malignant tumour (grey 'cells') growing amongst normal (white) cells of a tissue. Malignant tumours tend to grow by invasion (shown by arrows).

(g) The same malignant tumour shown in (f) has now grown a bit bigger and has invaded into the normal tissue around it.

An area of necrosis may develop in the middle of the tumour.

Normal cells in surrounding tissue

tumour

Normal cells in surrounding tissue less likely to be compressed by expanding tumour as it extends invasively between the cells.

Tumour cells may 'break away' from the main tumour mass (see *metastasis*, later).

tumour

Less likely that fibrous capsule forms at margin of tumour as there is less compression of normal cells.

On tissue surfaces, malignant tumours are more likely to be ulcerated or eroded (h), and therefore to bleed and get infected.

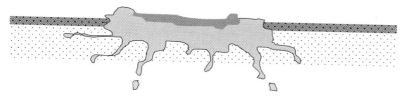

(h) A malignant tumour growing on the surface of a tissue or organ. There is central ulceration of the top surface of the tumour, and this can bleed and become infected.
Note that the tumour invades the normal tissues at its deep edges; these tumours can be difficult to dissect out at surgery, and the surgeon may take a wide margin of tissue which looks normal to try to ensure complete removal of the tumour.

Box 8.8 (*Continued*) Tumour growth patterns

With tubular or hollow organs, such as the intestine or bladder, tumours may grow around the inner surface of the wall (i). This is called annular growth, and when it is extensive it may cause blockage of the organ, leading to secondary disorders such as constipation or urine retention (depending on the organ affected). Annular growth can, in theory, occur with both benign and malignant tumours, but the malignant ones, which spread more readily, tend to cause most problems. The tumour in the organ wall may often ulcerate and bleed and so blood may be detected in the faeces, vomit or urine, and can be an indication of the presence of the tumour.

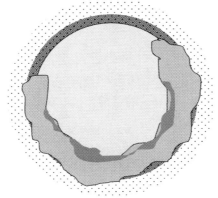

(i) Annular growth of a tumour in the wall of a hollow organ. Annular growth of a tumour may block the organ, and the tumour may ulcerate and bleed, and so blood may be detected in the faeces, vomit or urine, and can indicate the presence of the tumour.

Local invasion is not the same as spread to other areas or organs, which is the process known as metastasis. So, *metastasis* is the spread of malignant tumour from its site of origin (primary tumour) to form a secondary tumour which is also called a *metastasis* (plural *metastases*). Secondary tumours could themselves metastasise to form third stage or *tertiary* tumours though this is less common; unfortunately with many malignancies, the animal may not survive long enough for tertiary tumours to become established.

When considering treatment options for an animal with a tumour, it is common practice to take a radiograph or to scan areas such as the chest or liver to look for metastases before proceeding with treatment of the primary site. This procedure is often called a 'met check'.

There are a number of ways tumours can metastasise and these are discussed in the next section.

In order to metastasise, tumour cells require certain properties; they need to be able to move away from the main tumour site by interacting

Box 8.9 Metastasis of tumour cells via a vessel

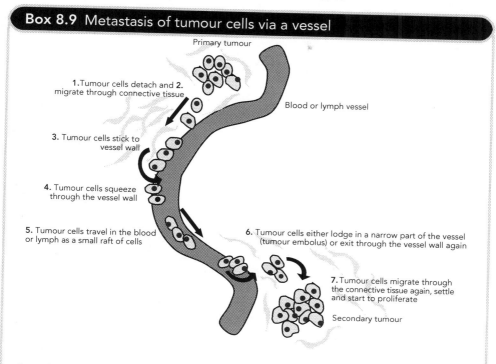

Primary tumour

1.Tumour cells detach and 2. migrate through connective tissue

Blood or lymph vessel

3. Tumour cells stick to vessel wall

4. Tumour cells squeeze through the vessel wall

5. Tumour cells travel in the blood or lymph as a small raft of cells

6. Tumour cells either lodge in a narrow part of the vessel (tumour embolus) or exit through the vessel wall again

7. Tumour cells migrate through the connective tissue again, settle and start to proliferate

Secondary tumour

In order to metastasise, tumour cells require to be able to perform certain tasks, illustrated in the cartoon.

1. They need to be able to move away from the main tumour site and to migrate by interacting with connective tissues **(2)**.

If they are going to use blood or lymph vessels to metastasise they need to stick to **(3.)** and then pass through the vessel walls **(4)**.

They need to travel in the blood or lymph and resist possible attack by the body's immune system **(5)**.

They may lodge in a narrow part of the vessel or they may need to adhere to and pass out through the vessel wall again **(6)**. Then they may need to migrate again through connective tissue at another site, and in another tissue type, to be able to establish at a new site **(7)** in order to form a secondary tumour.

Only a proportion of tumour cells are able successfully to pass all these tests, so metastasis is an inefficient business, and not all tumour cells which break away from the primary tumour site will form a secondary tumour.

with connective tissues; they may need to pass through blood or lymph vessel walls; they need to resist possible attack by the body's immune system, and they need to be able to establish at a new tissue site in order to proliferate and form a secondary tumour (Box 8.9). Only a proportion of tumour cells are able successfully to pass all these tests so metastasis is an inefficient business, and not all tumour cells which break away from the primary tumour site will lead to a secondary tumour mass.

Routes of metastasis

There are a number of possible ways for tumour cells to spread, discussed next (and summarised in Box 8.10). Tumours seem to have a preferred method of spread and some have preferred sites for their metastases to develop. For instance, metastases of prostate tumours in dogs will tend to establish in bone, whilst secondary malignant mammary tumours will usually occur in mammary lymph nodes.

- Metastasis via *haematogenous* spread: Haematogenous spread means spread of tumour cells via the blood circulatory system. This often also involves the lymphatic vessels since the lymph system drains into the blood vascular circulation. Haematogenous spread is mainly responsible for secondary tumours that grow in the liver, lungs and spleen.
- Metastasis via *lymphatic* spread: Lymph vessels are relatively 'easy' routes of spread for tumour cells. They are thin-walled and flow is under low pressure. When tumour cells enter lymphatic vessels near the primary tumour site, they travel to lymph nodes (which occur at intervals along the lymphatic circulation) and may establish a secondary tumour within the nodes. If the tumour cells are able to establish secondary tumours in nodes they will usually do so first in lymph nodes local to the primary tumour site. This is why vets will often seek out and sample local lymph nodes at the time of investigation of the primary tumour; the pathologist may be able to find tumour cells in the node and this can provide valuable prognostic information for the clinician and nurses. If tumour cells bypass the first lymph node they may still manage to entrap at more distant sites (so called *skip metastasis*), so absence of a secondary tumour in the first lymph node does not necessarily rule out metastatic spread of the primary tumour.

In many cases the lymph node will be enlarged if there is a secondary tumour within it. Note however that if the primary tumour is ulcerated and infected, its draining lymph nodes may well be enlarged because they are reacting to the infection rather than there necessarily being a secondary tumour present in the enlarged node.

- Metastasis via *serosal* spread: Another method of spread is by spread of tumour cells along serosal surfaces (or *serosae* – pronounced *ser-ro-zee*). Serosae are the slender tissue sheets or

Box 8.10 Summary of routes of metastasis of tumours

Haematogenous spread

- Spread of tumour cells via the blood circulatory system (may also involve lymphatic vessels since the lymph system drains into the blood circulation).
- Mainly involved in development of secondary tumours in the liver, lungs and spleen.

Lymphatic spread

- Spread of tumour cells in the lymph vessels.
- Lymph vessels are 'easy' routes of spread for tumour cells (thin walled, low pressure flow).
- Tumour cells entering lymphatic vessels near the primary tumour may spread first to a local lymph node and may establish a secondary tumour there.
- Local lymph nodes are often sampled at the time of investigation of the primary tumour to see whether the tumour has already spread.
- *Skip metastasis* is when tumour cells do not establish in the first lymph node but pass through it and form a secondary tumour at a more distant site. Thus, absence of a secondary tumour in the first lymph node does not rule out metastatic spread.
- An enlarged lymph node may mean there is a tumour in it. May also mean that there is infection of the primary tumour (especially if ulcerated) because infection and inflammatory cells will also be draining in the lymph from the primary tumour site to the local lymph node.

Serosal spread

- Spread of tumour cells along serosal surfaces (or *serosae*), such as peritoneum (covering abdominal organs), pleura (covering the lungs) and the epicardium of the heart.
- Sometimes called *serosal seeding* because neoplastic cells from tumours that form on/near serosal surfaces spread along the membranes like scattered seeds.
- These metastases stimulate the serosae to produce protein-rich fluid (exudate).
- Smears of fluid exudates from the abdomen or chest can be examined for presence of tumour cells.

Intra-organ spread

- Spread of tumour from one site in a particular organ to another site within the same organ.
- Uncommon means of tumour spread.
- May involve local surface 'seeding', e.g. along the inner lining surface of the trachea in the case of lung tumours, or may actually be via local blood or lymph drainage.

membranes that line body cavities and encase and suspend organs. Examples of serosae are the peritoneum which covers the abdominal organs, the pleural membranes which suspend the lungs and the epicardium of the heart. Neoplastic cells from tumours that form on or near the serosal surfaces are able to spread along the membranes like scattered seeds – so this method of tumour spread is sometimes called *serosal seeding*. These types of metastases often stimulate the serosae to produce a protein-rich fluid (exudate) which also contains free-floating tumour cells. Thus, fluid exudates from the abdomen or chest can be used diagnostically, when collected and examined as a smear under the microscope.

- Metastasis via *intra-organ* spread: As it sounds, intra-organ spread means spread of tumour from one site in a particular organ to another site within the same organ. This is an uncommon means of tumour spread and is thought to occur by various routes such as local surface 'seeding', e.g. along the inner lining surface of the trachea in the case of lung tumours, or via local blood or lymph drainage.

Note that not all malignant tumours do metastasise; some remain at their primary site and are locally invasive, though these can prove difficult to excise and often regrow at the site after surgery.

What effects do neoplasias have on the animal?

Physical presence of the tumour: Some effects of neoplasia on affected animals are simply due to the abnormal presence of a growing mass, and though many of the most harmful effects of tumours are associated with malignant masses, some benign tumours are harmful merely because of their position. So a tumour in the lungs may cause coughing or breathlessness, a mass in the stomach may stimulate vomiting whilst one in the urinary bladder may lead to inability to urinate. Brain tumours press on the brain as they grow within the rigid skull, adversely affecting brain function.

Bleeding and infection: Ulcerated, infected or highly vascular tumours, with a tendency to bleed easily, may provide additional clues to their presence because of blood, bacteria or inflammatory cells in sputum, vomit or urine.

Pain: Tumours may cause considerable pain due to pressure on or invasion into other organs; for instance, invasion of bone by tumour metastases is very painful.

Weight loss: Tumours are often associated with loss of body condition or wasting. This may be secondary to nausea, vomiting or inappetence. Marked wasting, known as cachexia, is also a primary effect of tumours and is due to the tumour secreting chemical messengers which increase breakdown of muscle (catabolic effects). Similar chemical messengers can lead to other non-specific signs such as fever (*pyrexia of unknown origin*, or PUO) or anaemia or leukopenia (decreased white blood cell count) due to inhibition of bone marrow.

Change in haematology: Ulcerated tumours of body surfaces can become infected, causing changes in the blood profile (increased neutrophils, for instance – see Chapter 4). In some cases the animal's response to the infection will be inhibited by effects of the tumour on the bone marrow. Blood clotting may also be adversely affected due to bone marrow inhibition, but also to any effects the tumour may have on liver function and decrease in clotting factors (see Chapter 7).

Inappropriate behaviour – increased or decreased hormone secretion: Many tumour cells still retain the functions of their normal cell of origin (see discussion of *differentiation*, earlier this chapter, page 165), but tend not to respond to normal control mechanisms.

In the case of tumours derived from a hormone-secreting cell of an endocrine organ for instance, the cells may secrete inappropriately high levels of hormone. Thus tumours of the pituitary gland of elderly dogs can lead to a form of *hyperadrenocorticism* or Cushing's disease. The tumour cells secrete adrenocorticotropic hormone (ACTH) which stimulates the cells of the adrenal cortex to produce cortisol. The tumour cells in the pituitary are resistant to the negative feedback mechanism that normally tones down their ACTH secretion when cortisol levels in the body reach a sufficient level. Stimulation of the adrenal glands continues unchecked producing the clinical signs of hyperadrenocorticism (Cushing's disease), such as altered metabolism, protein breakdown, impaired wound healing and reduced ability to mount an inflammatory response.

The opposite of hypersecretion by endocrinologically active (hormone-secreting) tumour cells is also occasionally found. In this case the tumour mass is composed of neoplastic cells that are not 'functionally active' (i.e. do not produce hormone at all). The growing mass of these inactive tumour cells presses on adjacent normal cells in the endocrine organ causing them to atrophy or die off (necrosis). Eventually, the function of the tissue is reduced because the inactive tumour cells take up more space than normal active endocrine cells. This so-called *space-occupying* effect is at least partially responsible for the complex effects of Cushing's disease in older horses. These horses have altered metabolism, deranged appetites and abnormal hair coats, and these changes are thought to be partially due to pressure of a growing pituitary tumour on the adjacent area of brain (the hypothalamus) which is responsible for regulation of body temperature, appetite and hair shedding.

Paraneoplastic syndromes: Another variation on this theme of secretion of substances by tumour cells is the secretion of substances *not normally* secreted by the cells which are making up the tumour. For instance, hormones may be secreted by tumour cells which are not actually of endocrine origin. This is the mechanism of a phenomenon called *paraneoplastic syndrome* (Box 8.11).

An example of this in veterinary medicine is encountered in some carcinomas of the anal sac and in some lymphomas. In these tumours, the neoplastic cells 'switch on' the ability to secrete a substance closely related to parathyroid hormone (PTH) which is normally produced by the parathyroid glands. Normal PTH acts to increase blood calcium levels partly by encouraging release of calcium from bone. It does this by stimulating large cells called osteoclasts which are related to macrophages and which nibble away at the bone's surface and release calcium into the bloodstream. The impostor hormone, produced by the neoplastic cells, is called parathyroid-related peptide or PThRP for short. PThRP acts in the same way as PTH and a marked and inappropriately high blood calcium level (*hypercalcaemia*) can be a diagnostic sign for these two tumours (see Box 8.12).

The immune system and neoplasia

It is known that incidence of malignant tumours of some types increases in animals with poor immune systems (*immunocompromised* animals). So, could it be that other animals with adequate immune function are able to make an immune response, and limit the development of these malignancies?

When viewed under the microscope, some tumours are surrounded by clusters of lymphocytes (these cells are associated with immune responses – see Chapter 5). In some of these cases an apparent response by the immune system is associated with better prognosis and even with reduction in size (regression) of tumours.

An example of immune-mediated regression of a tumour is the cutaneous histiocytoma, a skin tumour common in young dogs. These tumours are often excised and sent to a pathology laboratory to confirm the diagnosis. Under the microscope, clusters of lymphocytes are often present at the edges of these tumours and, if not surgically removed, most simple benign histiocytomas would eventually be destroyed by the immune system. The possibility of a role of the immune system in tumour regression suggests that effective vaccines against certain tumour types will be developed in the future.

Another example of the immune response fighting tumours, encouraged by vaccination, is with tumours known to be caused by a virus.

Box 8.11 Paraneoplastic syndrome: inappropriate production of a hormone or substance which mimics a normal hormone

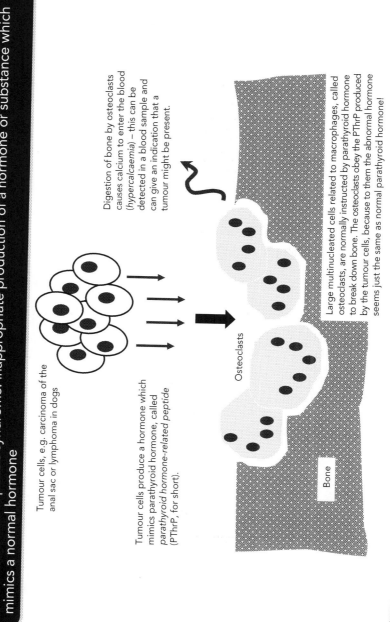

Tumour cells, e.g. carcinoma of the anal sac or lymphoma in dogs

Tumour cells produce a hormone which mimics parathyroid hormone, called *parathyroid hormone-related peptide* (PThrP, for short).

Osteoclasts

Bone

Digestion of bone by osteoclasts causes calcium to enter the blood (*hypercalcaemia*) – this can be detected in a blood sample and can give an indication that a tumour might be present.

Large multinucleated cells related to macrophages, called osteoclasts, are normally instructed by parathyroid hormone to break down bone. The osteoclasts obey the PThrP produced by the tumour cells, because to them the abnormal hormone seems just the same as normal parathyroid hormone!

Box 8.12 Summary of the effects of tumours

Physical presence of the tumour	• Abnormal presence of a growing mass compresses normal tissues or causes blockages of hollow organs.
Bleeding and infection	• Ulcerated, infected or highly vascular tumours, with a tendency to bleed easily, may shed blood, bacteria or inflammatory cells in sputum, vomit or urine.
Pain	• Due to pressure on or invasion into other organs, e.g. invasion of bone by tumour metastases is very painful.
Weight loss	• May be secondary to nausea, vomiting or inappetence. • Tumour *cachexia* (marked wasting) is also due to the tumour secreting chemical messengers which increase metabolic breakdown of muscle.
Non-specific signs due to chemical messengers secreted by tumour cells	• Such as fever (PUO), and anaemia or leukopenia (decreased white blood cell count) due to inhibition of bone marrow.
Change in haematology	• Ulcerated tumours can become infected, causing changes in the blood (e.g. increased neutrophils). • Inflammatory response may be inhibited by inhibitory effects of the tumour on bone marrow. • Blood clotting may also be adversely affected due to bone marrow inhibition, also to the effects the tumour may have on liver function and decreased clotting factors.
Inappropriate behaviour, i.e. increased or decreased hormone secretion	• Many tumour cells retain the functions of their normal cell of origin but tend not to respond to normal control mechanisms. • In the case of tumours derived from hormone-secreting (endocrine) organs, the cells may secrete inappropriately high levels of hormone. • Alternatively, endocrine tumours may be composed of neoplastic cells that do not produce hormone. The growing tumour presses on adjacent normal cells in the endocrine organ causing atrophy or necrosis. The function of the endocrine organ is reduced as a result.
Paraneoplastic syndromes	• Secretion of substances *not normally* secreted by the cells from which the tumour forms, e.g. hormones may be secreted by tumour cells which are not of endocrine origin (Box 8.11).

These tumours could be prevented by vaccinations specifically against the virus. The vaccine aims to ensure that the host's own immune system fights off the virus when the host is exposed to it, and therefore the tumours will not (or are less likely to) develop. An example of this is feline leukaemia virus (FeLV) vaccination, and in human medicine a vaccine against human papilloma virus (HPV), intended to prevent cervical cancers, has recently been developed.

This is a rapidly developing area, but the intriguing possibility of control or treatment of neoplasia by vaccination is likely to receive considerable attention in the future.

Diagnosis of neoplasms in veterinary general practice

Not so long ago it was sufficient to find out whether a tumour in an animal was benign, in which case the prognosis was likely to be good, or malignant, in which case it was not. Nowadays, advances in our understanding of tumour development, with increased availability of specific treatments, and owners prepared to try treatment for their pets, means that precise diagnosis of tumours is more important.

Primary assessment of a tumour patient is likely to start with clinical examination and include blood and urine sampling and radiography, as appropriate.

Depending on interest and experience in the practice, *cytology* may be used to try to make a diagnosis or to investigate whether the tumour has spread to another site. Cytological techniques used in general practice are thin smears on glass microscope slides of samples such as fine-needle aspirates (FNAs), which may be gently sucked with a syringe (aspirated) from the middle of the tumour. FNAs may also be made from fluids such as bronchiolar lavage (BAL – washed from the trachea), urine or peritoneal tap fluids. Finally, a tumour or part of a tumour may be dabbed on to the glass slide to produce impression smears of tissues. All these preparations may be air-dried, stained and examined under the microscope in the practice laboratory. Alternatively, the dried slides may be sent to a pathology laboratory so that the clinical pathologist can examine them.

Cytology is a useful early step in diagnosis, being relatively cheap, easy and non-invasive (compared with biopsy). Good quality smears are useful for assessing some of the cell features included in Box 8.14 and may allow rapid diagnosis or at least might indicate that further procedures (such as biopsy) are warranted.

The next step is examination of tissue (histology) rather than smears of cells (cytology). Histology involves microscopic examination by a pathologist, of formalin-fixed tissues collected at surgery (biopsy). (See

Box 8.13 Useful information for the pathologist

When you send any formalin-fixed tissue (biopsy) to the laboratory for histology (in addition to clinical history, signs and signalment) note down:

- Site of tumour(s)
- How long the tumour(s) took to develop
- Measurements (approximate are better than nothing!)
- Other features, e.g. describe ulceration, haemorrhage
- Evaluate and comment upon local invasion if possible/appropriate
- Evaluate and comment upon attachment to surrounding tissues (or comment on how easy it was to remove – 'shell out')
- Evaluate and comment upon local lymph node involvement (if possible)
- If there is more than one tumour – examine, describe and sample as many as possible
- Include and comment upon imaging results (radiography, scan results etc.)

Chapter 1 for information on how the formalin-fixed specimen ends up under the pathologist's microscope.)

An *incisional* biopsy is when a part (a slice or a needle core) is removed and fixed. An *excisional* biopsy, on the other hand, is the term used when the entire mass has been removed and fixed. If the removed specimen is large it is best to cut it into smaller pieces to allow the formalin to penetrate before you send it to the laboratory. If this is not done, the centre of the specimen will not fix properly and may start to deteriorate (*autolyse*) on the way to the laboratory.

In order to offer a diagnosis, the pathologist interprets cell features of the neoplastic cells, but also assesses relationships of the tumour cells to normal tissue and looks for signs of invasion of the tumour. The practice must send some paperwork with the tissue, in order to provide the pathologist with useful information to help reach a diagnosis. As well as the clinical history and signalment of the animal it is really helpful for the pathologist to have information about the tumour(s) and any other relevant information which may help (Box 8.13). The pathologist will assess histological features such as those summarised in Box 8.14. In addition, the pathologist may be able to indicate whether the mass has been removed entirely by commenting on the *excision margins*. The excision margins are the amount of normal tissue surrounding the tumour on the microscope slide. The pathologist may be able to find microscopic evidence of local invasion of tumour cells into adjacent tissues, which may not have been apparent when the specimen was examined grossly. In some cases the vet may then decide it is worth performing more surgery to remove a little more tissue from the previous surgery site, ensuring *clean* excision margins (free of tumour cells).

Box 8.14 The histological features of benign versus malignant tumours

Benign tumour cells (or low grade malignancy)
- Cells and nuclei are relatively uniform (look like cells of origin)

- Mitotic index* – may be low or high
- Uniform mitotic figures¶

- Arrangement of tumour cells may look similar to the normal tissue of origin (recognisable tissue architecture)
- No indication of invasion of adjacent tissue

Malignant cells
- Cells and nuclei are non-uniform (tissue of origin may be not be clear) (see photographs in Box 8.15)
- Mitotic index* – may be low or high
- Abnormal or irregular mitotic figures (see photographs in Box 8.15)
- Tumour usually does not retain recognisable tissue architecture

- Invasion of adjacent tissues and/or vessels (see photographs in Box 8.15)
- Tumour cells in other tissues (e.g. local lymph node)
- Necrosis within tumour

* *Mitotic index* is a count of the number of cells seen to be dividing by mitosis (or the number of mitotic figures). For instance, an average of the counts of mitoses per ten high power views under the microscope of the tumour is given as the mitotic index.

¶ *Mitotic figures* are made up of the separating nuclear material of cells undergoing division by mitosis. They appear under the microscope as two equal-sized densely staining frilly bands in normal cell divisions. In abnormal divisions the nuclear material divides unequally or appears in strange forms, like 'Y' or 'X' shapes, or even stranger arrangements (Box 8.15).

Sometimes, especially if cells appear very abnormal under the microscope, a diagnosis is not able to be made by standard histology. The pathologist and the vet may decide to use more specialist techniques to make the diagnosis. These techniques include an extremely high-powered microscope called an electron microscope, or immuno-histochemistry (discussed next).

Immunohistochemistry

This is very specific staining based on immune reactions. Solutions of antibodies to specific cell proteins (that is particular proteins normally occurring in or on certain cells – *antigens*, see Chapter 5) are applied to the tissue section on a microscope slide. The antibodies are labelled with a colour (usually brown) which can be seen under the microscope and they attach themselves to their specific target protein. If antibodies to tumour cells suspected of being present are used then this technique will confirm a presumptive diagnosis. In this way the pathologist can recognise very specific cell types, and can say more accurately what sort of tumour is present.

Box 8.15 Photographs of normal and abnormal mitoses

Mitotic figures

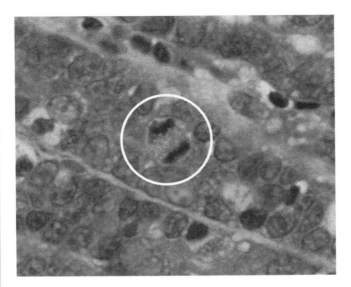

(a) Above, normal mitotic figure (circled) in a dividing epithelial cells in the gut. Two pretty much equal sets of nuclear material are seen as two dark bands in the cell. They are drawing apart and when the cell divides, each new cell will get an equal share of the nuclear material.

(b) Below, an abnormal or bizarre mitotic figure in a malignant tumour on a dog's leg. There has been very uneven division of nuclear material, with one large irregular main band and several small blobs of nuclear material beside this.

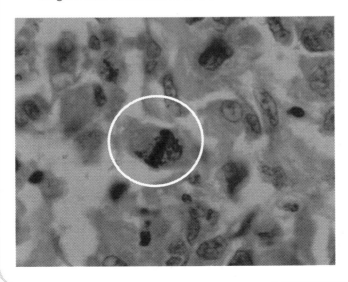

Box 8.15 *(Continued)* Photographs of abnormal cellular features and metastasising neoplastic cells

Neoplastic cells may have abnormal cell shapes and sizes

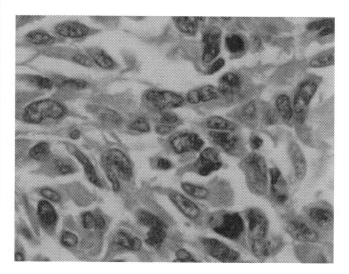

(c) Above, nuclei of tumour cells in this photograph from the same tumour as shown in (b) are very irregular in shape, size and appearance. Some cells have more than one nucleus.

(d) Below, a 'raft' or micrometastasis of tumour cells in a blood vessel from a malignant tumour in a horse's foot. You can spot irregular nuclei of a some loose tumour cells amongst the red blood cells too.

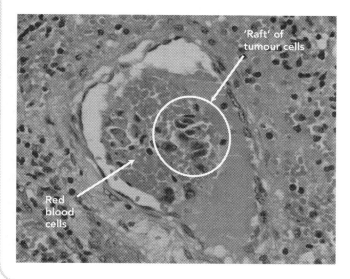

In the future, it is likely that more techniques will be developed for the investigation of tumours in veterinary practice. For instance, the medical profession are already making use of substances known as *tumour markers* which are secreted into the bloodstream by tumour cells and are discussed next.

Tumour markers

Tumour markers are a relatively non-invasive indication of the presence or the regrowth of tumours, requiring collection of blood samples by standard methods. An example of their use is in men to detect or to monitor prostate cancer. Detection of the marker, known as *prostate-specific antigen* (PSA), in blood samples provides a potential screening test for early detection of the disease before clinical signs start. Furthermore, reappearance of the marker some time after surgical removal of the tumour can indicate that the tumour has regrown.

It is possible that tumour markers will become used in veterinary medicine, as research has so far included their investigation in various tumours in dogs including prostate tumours, and tumours of liver, biliary tract, pancreas and testes.

In conclusion, we now have a far greater understanding of how neoplasms (tumours) develop in men and animals, including the specific causes and mechanisms of cell transformation for numerous tumour types. There are newer, sometimes more reliable and sophisticated methods of diagnosing neoplasia and treating cancers. In many cases treatments are able to spare normal cells and target *only* the neoplastic ones. Owners also have greater knowledge and experience; additionally, they may pay into insurance schemes, or for various other reasons be more inclined to opt for treatment –perhaps at a specialist centre – when previously they might not have wished to proceed.

Oncology, the study of neoplasms and their development, is a rapidly expanding field. Even if you are working in a first opinion practice, from which animals are referred to specialist centres for treatment, worried owners may need to discuss their animal with you and they may have special nursing requirements when the animal returns from treatment sessions, or they may just require advice on what to expect. It will certainly help you, them and their pets if you keep up to date with the scientific advances and treatments, and nursing techniques, for animals with neoplasia.

Summary of key points in Chapter 8

- Atrophy, hypertrophy, hyperplasia and metaplasia are reversible adaptive changes in cells which help the cell to cope with an alteration in its environment.
- *Atrophy* is *shrinkage* in the size of cells (and therefore the tissue of which the cell forms part) in response to a stimulus. There are a number of causes of atrophy.
- *Hypertrophy* is *increase in size* of cells in response to a stimulus, whereas *hyperplasia* is *increase in the number* of cells. Sometimes both processes occur together.
- *Metaplasia* is conversion of one mature cell type to another.
- *Neoplasia* is an irreversible cell change. It involves the proliferation of *abnormal* cells to form *neoplasms* (cancers or tumours). Unlike the reversible changes, neoplastic cells cannot revert to normal once the stimulus is removed.
- Neoplastic changes (*transformations*) are genetic mutations and are passed on to new cells when the neoplastic cell divides. All tumours therefore originate from one transformed cell. Neoplastic cells grow and divide in an uncontrolled manner.
- Metastasis is the process of spread of tumour cells to form secondary tumours (metastases). There are various routes of metastasis.
- Neoplasms have various direct and indirect harmful effects on animals. It may be that the immune response could be manipulated to fight certain tumours.
- There are various clinical and pathological diagnostic techniques for recognising tumours and for making a prognosis.

Test yourself questions on Chapter 8

1. a. List four common reversible cell adaptations /changes involving altered cell growth or size
   b. Construct a simple diagram to illustrate the changes you have named in part 1.a.
   c. Define neoplasia, and indicate what fundamental way neoplasia differs from the changes you listed in part 1.a.
2. a. Stages of changes to the genetic make-up of a cell are fundamental to tumour development, name the three stages of genetic abnormality that are recognised in the development of tumours.
   b. A factor able to cause permanent DNA damage and thus lead to tumour formation is called a carcinogen. List some groups of carcinogenic factors for domestic animals.
3. Draw up a simple table outlining the most common differences between benign and malignant tumours
4. a. What is meant by the term *metastasis*?
   b. Name three means by which tumours metastasise.
5. Make short notes to discuss two of the ways a tumour exerts harmful effects on an animal.
6. Discuss cytology in the diagnosis of neoplasms in veterinary general practice.

Glossary

This glossary is a quick reference list of terms used in this book, plus a few extra ones that you may come across in your further reading, with definitions. It is not meant to be a comprehensive medical dictionary, but is a list of words likely to be helpful in your understanding of general pathology.

Most of the following terms appear in italics when you encounter them elsewhere in this book. There is cross-reference between terms in this glossary too, also indicated by words in italics.

Abscess A localised accumulation of pus, often with a fibrous wall around it, which is the result of an inflammatory reaction, especially where bacteria and necrosis are involved. See *pus* and *suppuration*.

Acquired diseases Diseases that develop at some stage during life, as a result of the effects of one or more aetiological agent acting during life. See also *aetiology* and *aetiological agent*.

Acquired immune system/response Specific defence mechanisms in the body against infectious agents and other foreign molecules. See *adaptive immune system/response*.

Acute inflammation Rapidly developing inflammation, usually of relatively short duration, and characterised by blood vessel dilation and leakiness (oedema) and by influx of neutrophils. See also *inflammation* and *chronic inflammation*.

Adaptive immune system/response A defensive system in the body which is specifically stimulated to respond by infectious agents and other foreign molecules. Responses are *cellular*, involving T *lymphocytes* and *macrophages*, or are *humoral*, involving the production of *antibodies* (*immunoglobulins*) by activated B lymphocytes. Also known as *acquired* or *specific* immunity.

Adenocarcinoma A malignant tumour formed from glandular cells, such as mammary gland cells. See also *carcinoma* and *sarcoma*.

Aetiological agent A factor capable of causing disease. See also *aetiology*, *pathogen* and *pathogenic*.

Aetiology The study of the causes of disease.

Allergy Also known as type I or immediate hypersensitivity. An immune response involving release of active substances by stimulated mast cells in response to an *antigen* (see below). See also *anaphylaxis*.

Anaemia Abnormally low haemoglobin or red blood cell level in the blood, which affects the oxygen carrying function of the blood.

Anaphylactic shock Severe acute fall in blood pressure due to extreme hypersensitivity of an animal. Something to which the animal is sensitive (the allergen) stimulates marked mast cell degranulation. The contents of the released mast cell granules stimulate dilation of blood vessels which causes the sudden decrease in blood pressure.

See also *allergy, anaphylaxis, hypersensitivity, shock, cardiogenic shock, hypovolaemic shock, neurogenic shock, toxic shock, septic shock* and *types I–IV hypersensitivity reactions.*

Anaphylaxis   A very sudden severe, maybe life-threatening, immediate allergic or type I hypersensitivity reaction to a stimulus to which the host is especially sensitive.

Anasarca   Generalised accumulation of tissue fluid all over the body. See also *ascites, oedema, hydropericardium, hydrothorax* and *hydroperitoneum.*

Anatomic pathology   Pathology which involves the examination of tissues or organs. This may involve post-mortem examinations (also called *necropsies*) or looking at tissues from live animals (called *biopsies*). Anatomic pathologists look at the tissues or organs by eye (gross examination) to identify abnormalities, but also use histologic sections mounted on glass slides and stained, to examine the tissue under the microscope.

Antibodies   Special proteins produced by certain cells of the body's immune system in response to a foreign *antigen* (see below). Also known as *immunoglobulins*. Antibody production is part of what is known as the *immune response*. See also *plasma cells.*

Antibody complexes   Clumps of *antigen* and *antibody* which form in most immune responses. The complexes attract the proteins of the *complement* cascade and are usually ultimately destroyed by *phagocytic* cells. See also *type III hypersensitivity.*

Antigen   Any foreign substance (such as an infectious organism) that can stimulate an immune response in the host. See also *antigenicity* and *blood groups.*

Antigenicity   The tendency for a foreign substance (such as an infectious agent) to be recognised by an antibody or lymphocyte and to provoke an immune response.

Apoptosis   A form of cell death that is caused by release of protein-digesting enzymes within the cell. Apoptosis occurs under both normal and pathological conditions. For instance, it is involved in normal 'modelling' of the growing embryo, but also in the removal (by death) of cells infected by some viruses. Apoptosis is distinct from *necrosis.*

Ascites   Abnormal accumulation of fluid within the abdomen. See also *oedema.*

Atrophy   When cells within a tissue shrink, causing the whole organ composed of those cells to decrease in size.

Autoimmune disease   A disease which results when the immune system attacks the body's own tissues.

Autolysis   Literally means the splitting (or breaking up) of self. Refers to cells being digested by enzymes contained within their cytoplasm (in vesicles called *lysosomes*). Usually used in the context of death of cells in a body after death, i.e. post-mortem decomposition. See also *lysosomes* and *necrosis*.

Bacteraemia   Bacteria circulating in the blood. See also *septicaemia*.

Basophil   A cell with a segmented nucleus and intracytoplasmic granules (which stain blue in histological sections). Basophils take part in allergic or type I (immediate) hypersensitivity reactions. See also *allergy* and *type I/immediate hypersensitivity*.

Benign tumour   A tumour which is usually well-demarcated and does not spread (by *metastasis*). See also *neoplasia* and *malignant tumour*.

Biopsy   Specimen from a live animal (such as a tumour, a skin lesion, or a piece of an internal organ) which is fixed in formalin and sent to a pathologist for a histopathological diagnosis. Biopsies may be of various sizes, and may include all or only part of a lesion of tissue). See also *pinch biopsy*, *punch biopsy*, *incisional biopsy* and *excisional biopsy*.

Blood coagulation   Clotting of the blood protein *fibrin* and *platelets*. See *coagulation*.

Blood groups   Proteins of a certain type, which are on the surface of red blood cells. If red blood cells bearing one type of protein are injected into a host whose red blood cells carry a different protein (i.e. the host is of another blood group), then the proteins of the injected cells act as *antigens*. An immune response against the injected cells ensues and they are destroyed. This is the basis of transfusion reactions when donor and recipient are not matched in terms of blood group. See also *antigen* and *antigenicity*.

Calcification   Normal in some tissues (bones or teeth), but also refers to abnormal deposition of hard calcium in disease or in damaged tissues ('*dystrophic*' *calcification*) or when the level of calcium in the blood is abnormally high ('*metastatic*' *calcification*).

Carcinogen   An agent (often refers to a chemical) capable of causing tumours to develop in animals exposed to that agent.

Carcinogenesis   The mechanisms and processes of tumour development in the body. See also *oncogenesis* which may be used interchangeably with carcinogenesis.

Carcinoma   A malignant tumour (neoplasm) originating from cells of epithelial type, that is cells of body surfaces. See also *sarcoma*.

Cardiogenic shock   Sudden potentially life-threatening fall in blood pressure due to acute heart failure. The failed heart is suddenly unable to pump blood effectively and this causes a marked decrease in cardiac output. See also *shock*, *anaphylactic shock*, *hypovolaemic shock*, *neurogenic shock*, *toxic shock* and *septic shock*.

Caseation necrosis   A type of cell necrosis characterised by the dead tissue acquiring a cheesy consistency with loss of normal cellular and organ architecture. See also *necrosis, coagulative necrosis, liquefactive necrosis, fat necrosis, gangrene, wet gangrene, dry gangrene* and *gas gangrene.*

Cell-mediated immunity/immune response   An immune response involving lymphocytes and macrophages, rather than *antibodies.* See also *humoral immunity.*

Cellular degeneration   *Reversible cell damage,* from which the cell can recover if the damaging stimulus is removed. See also *cloudy swelling, irreversible cell damage* and *necrosis.*

Cellulitis   Inflammation in connective tissue.

Chemical pathology   The type of pathology used in the laboratory. See *clinical pathology.*

Cholestasis   Stoppage of the flow of bile in the biliary tract; may result in *jaundice.*

Chronic inflammation   Slowly developing or long-lasting inflammation, usually involving *macrophages* and proliferation of fibrous tissue. See also *inflammation* and *acute inflammation.*

Clinical pathology   The type of pathology used in the laboratory, whether a practice laboratory or a diagnostic laboratory. For instance, urinalysis or blood biochemistry are clinical or chemical pathology techniques. Clinical pathologists assess disease in an animal by studying body fluids (such as blood, urine, joint fluid, abdominal tap fluid, cerebro-spinal fluid and so on) or by microscopic examination of stained cells from the fluids, or from *fine-needle aspirates* (FNAs). See also *cytology* and *general pathology* for contrast.

Cloudy swelling   Early stage of reversible cell damage (see *cellular degeneration*), in which the cell swells with water and the cytoplasm becomes pale. See also *reversible* and *irreversible cell damage* and *necrosis.*

Coagulation (of blood)   The clotting of blood as a result of the activation of a series of proteins, which forms a *fibrin* clot and coats *platelets* (and other cells). Blood coagulation is meant to be a safety mechanism to prevent leakage of blood from the circulation in the event of blood vessel damage. In some instances, however, it can occur inappropriately and be harmful. See also *consumption coagulopathy, disseminated intravascular coagulation, haemorrhage* and *thrombus.*

Coagulative necrosis   A form of cell death (necrosis) in which the cell contents become coagulated and form an amorphous mass, but the cell's outline (basic architecture) is retained. See also *necrosis, caseation necrosis, liquefactive necrosis, fat necrosis, gangrene, wet gangrene, dry gangrene, moist gangrene* and *gas gangrene.*

Coagulopathy   General term meaning a disease affecting the blood clotting system; it is usually used in connection with diseases which result in decreased clotting ability (bleeding tendency). See also *consumption coagulopathy*, *disseminated intravascular coagulation* and *haemorrhage*.

Collagen   A firm fibrous protein, stronger and more permanent than *fibrin*, and produced by cells called fibroblasts in the connective tissue of the body. See also *fibrin* and *fibroblasts*.

Collagenous   Fibrous tissue contains lots of *collagen* and is said to be *collagenous*. See also *fibrin* and *fibroblasts*.

Complement   A cascade of serum proteins activated by the process of *antibody* binding to *antigen*, and which results in cells being destroyed or by clumping of bacteria or other foreign substances.

Congenital disease/condition   A condition present at birth that has been caused by something which happened to the developing embryo or foetus before birth. Congenital conditions are not necessarily hereditary (able to be passed on to the offspring of the affected animal). See *hereditary disease/condition* and *genetic disease/condition*.

Consumption coagulopathy   When haemorrhages occur as a result of clotting factors being used up (consumed) due to another process, such as widespread clotting (see *disseminated intravascular coagulation*). Note that consumed or consumption in this case is not connected with eating something (oral consumption) so is not referring to the animal eating a poison such as rat poison, for instance. Consumed/consumption have alternative meanings connected with something being 'used up'; it is this meaning that is relevant in this context.

Crepitus   Used to describe the feel of fractured bone fragments rubbing together, also the feel of gas in tissues, such as occurs in *gas gangrene*.

Cytokine   Chemical messengers produced by various cell types, which are important in cell-to-cell communication in immune responses and in inflammation.

Cytology   Examination of cells in body fluid or in a *fine-needle aspirate*, by use of a microscope to study a stained smear of the sample on a glass microscope slide.

Cytotoxic   This is a broad term meaning harmful or lethal to cells. Note that, despite its sound, the term is not used solely in reference to *toxins*, for instance, there is a class of the immune cells *T lymphocytes* known as cytotoxic lymphocytes.

Cytotoxic hypersensitivity   Also known as *type II hypersensitivity reaction*. An immune response in which elements of the immune system are directed to kill cells of the body because the target cells have been inappropriately coated with *antibodies*.

Degranulation   The release of the active contents of granules in the cytoplasm of cells such as *neutrophils, mast cells* and *eosinophils* when the cells are activated.

Delayed type hypersensitivity   Also known as *type IV hypersensitivity*. An inflammatory response, involving cells of the immune system, which can take several hours (24–72 hours) to develop after the animal is exposed to the stimulus to which that animal is sensitive.

Dendritic cells   Large, long-lived cells with cellular processes (arms), that act as antigen-presenting cells. That is to say, they pick up *antigen* in the tissues, carry it back to the lymphoid organs and then 'hold it out' for recognition by *lymphocytes* called T cells, in order to stimulate an *immune response*.

Disseminated   Widespread or diffuse in the body.

Disseminated intravascular coagulation (DIC)   A serious, usually fatal, condition in which there is diffuse activation of the blood clotting mechanism throughout the blood circulation of a live animal. As a result, clotting factors may be used up (consumed) and so widespread small haemorrhages may ensue secondarily. See also *coagulopathy* and *consumption coagulopathy*.

Dry gangrene   A type of tissue death due to loss of blood supply. No bacteria are involved. The tissue feels cold, dry and shrivelled, and is discoloured. See also *gangrene, gas gangrene, moist gangrene* and *wet gangrene*.

Dystrophic calcification   Abnormal deposition of hard calcium in disease or in damaged tissues. See also *calcification* and *metastatic calcification*.

Ecchymoses   Discrete haemorrhages in the skin or within (or on) organs, larger than *petechiae*. See also *haemorrhage, petechiae* and *haematoma*.

Effusion   An abnormal accumulation of fluid in a body cavity or area.

Embolus   A substance (fluid, solid or gas) which is able to lodge in a blood vessel and cause a blockage. See also *infarction, ischaemia, thrombus* and *thrombosis*.

Endogenous   Refers to something formed, produced or acting from within the body (or cell). For instance, endogenous glucocorticoids are produced by the adrenal glands. The opposite of *exogenous*.

Endothelium   The lining layer of blood and lymph vessels formed by a thin single layer of flattened (endothelial) cells.

Eosinophil   A white blood cell with a complex segmented (or lobed) nucleus (i.e. not a single rounded nucleus, like a *macrophage*). Eosinophils have granules in their cytoplasm and the contents of the granules are released when the cells are activated. Eosinophils are often associated with parasite infections or with allergies or sensitivities.

Erosion   Partial loss of the surface layer of an organ or tissue, for instance, gastric erosion or erosion of the skin. See also *ulcer*.

Excision margins   An assessment by the pathologist of the amount of normal tissue included around the edge of a biopsy of a lesion, usually a tumour. If the pathologist suggests that excision margins are adequate or good then the tumour may have been completely removed. If, on the other hand, the pathologist comments that excision margins are narrow or that tumour cells extend to the edge of the specimen, then further surgery at the site may be required to try to remove remaining tumour cells, and stop the tumour regrowing at that site.

Excisional biopsy   Removal of a pathological lesion (such as a tumour or ulcer), usually with some surrounding normal tissue. This is fixed and sent to the pathologist for examination. See also *excision margins* and *incisional biopsy*.

Exogenous   Refers to something formed, produced in or acting from outside the body (or cell). For instance, exogenous glucocorticoids are given as corticosteroid injections, though the body also produces steroids (see also *endogenous*).

Exudate   Accumulation of protein-rich fluid due to leakiness of blood vessels, for instance, inflammatory exudate. See also *transudate*.

Fatty change   The accumulation of lipid (fat) in the cytoplasm of cells; a *reversible cell change*. See also *cloudy swelling* and *cellular degeneration*.

Fibrin   A protein formed by the activation of fibrinogen. Fibrin tends to form a soft gel-like mass, which plugs wounds or damaged areas of endothelium and forms the foundation of blood clots or wound healing.

Fibrinogen   A soluble protein in the blood plasma which is converted to *fibrin* (gel-like clots of insoluble protein) in the processes of clotting or tissue repair.

Fibrosis   The formation of the strong fibrous protein, collagen, usually as part of the scar process when badly damaged tissues heal. See also *organisation* and *tissue repair*.

Gangrene   A variant of coagulative necrosis. Gangrene is the necrosis that occurs due to loss of blood supply to an area, especially an extremity. The affected part is cold to touch. Four types of gangrene are described, *dry, gas, moist* and *wet*.

Gas gangrene   A type of tissue death due to loss of blood supply. In this form of gangrene, gas-producing bacteria proliferate in the necrotic tissue. The affected tissue has a crackly (crepitant) feel. See also *gangrene, dry gangrene, moist gangrene, wet gangrene* and *crepitus.*

General pathology   The study of the basic pathological processes that are not specific to particular organs or tissues. For instance, processes such as cell degeneration, inflammation and tumour formation are similar in all parts of the body, and so are considered under the heading of general pathology.

Genes   Segments of chromosomes, genes are made up of deoxyribonucleic acid (DNA). Each gene contains the information for a particular physical or functional characteristic of the cell. All cells contain all the genetic information of the animal, but not all genes will be functional in every cell all of the time.

Genetic disease/condition   A disease caused by an abnormality in the genes of an animal. This abnormality may be passed on to the offspring. See *hereditary condition* or *disease.*

Globulins   A group of soluble proteins in blood serum; includes the *immunoglobulins.* See *antibodies.*

Granulation tissue   A type of soft spongy connective tissue which forms early in the process of tissue healing. Granulation tissue contains cells which produce collagen fibres, capillaries, and inflammatory cells. Note that granulation tissue is *not* the same thing as *granulomatous inflammation.* See also *organisation.*

Granuloma   A specific arrangement of inflammatory cells, principally *macrophages,* which can occur in certain types of chronic inflammation. See also *granulomatous inflammation.*

Granulomatous inflammation   Granulomatous inflammation is a form of chronic inflammation which primarily involves *macrophages,* though sometimes other cell types (such as *plasma cells* and *lymphocytes*) help out. Often the inflammatory cells are arranged in *granulomas.* Note that granulomatous inflammation is not the same thing as *granulation tissue.*

Haematocrit   The proportion of blood which is composed of cells. The haematocrit varies under certain physiological or pathological conditions. For instance, dehydration will increase the haematocrit. See also *haemoconcentration.*

Haematology   Specifically the study of cell types in blood. For instance, haematology can indicate an increase in white blood cells (*leucocytes*) in an animal fighting an infection or a decrease in red blood cells (*erythrocytes*) in an animal with anaemia.

Haematoma   A type of localised haemorrhage, usually within a solid organ or tissue, e.g. aural haematoma, or bruising within muscle. See also *haemorrhage, ecchymoses* and *petechiae.*

Haemoconcentration   An increase in the proportion of cells in the blood due to a decrease in the fluid content. See also *haematocrit.*

Haemolysis Destruction of red blood cells often due to an inappropriate immune response to the red cells. See also *blood groups*.

Haemopericardium, haemothorax, haemoperitoneum The prefix *haemo-* indicates haemorrhage into the area indicated, in these instances into the pericardial sac (around the heart), into the thorax and into the peritoneal cavity (around the abdominal organs).

Haemorrhage Escape of blood from the blood vascular system. See also *haematoma*, *ecchymoses* and *petechiae*.

Hereditary disease or condition A disorder that can be passed on from either or both parents to their offspring. More than one offspring may be affected, or successive offspring may have the disease.

Histamine A potent biological chemical, which is produced by *mast cells*. Histamine has a number of actions, including the ability to stimulate *endothelial* cell contraction, which opens up gaps between the cells in the capillary walls, thus allowing the escape of protein-rich *exudate* into surrounding tissues. Histamine is also able to cause vasodilation. See also *acute inflammation* and *type I hypersensitivity*.

Histopathology The examination under the microscope of tissues from a diseased animal or from a specific lesion. The tissues are fixed (e.g. in formalin) or frozen, processed, cut into a very thin section and mounted on a glass slide. They must then be stained to make the cells show up more clearly when examined microscopically.

Humoral immunity/immune response That part of the immune response which is dependent on *antibodies*, rather than the action of cells of the immune system. See also *cell-mediated immunity*.

Hydropericardium, hydrothorax The prefix *hydro-* indicates accumulation of fluid in the area indicated, in these instances in the pericardial sac (around the heart) and in the thorax. See also *ascites* and *oedema*.

Hydrostatic pressure Literally, water pressure. In blood vessels the hydrostatic pressure of the blood normally tends to push fluid out into the tissue (*interstitium*) from the capillaries. See also *osmotic pressure*.

Hyperaemia An increased blood flow to an area, usually due to increased flow through a dilated capillary bed. The area becomes hot and reddened as a result, such as in *acute inflammation*.

Hypercoagulability In blood, the increased tendency to clot. See also *Virchow's triad*.

Hyperplasia Enlargement of an organ due to an increase in the number of its cells. See also *hypertrophy*.

Hypersensitivity An inappropriate inflammatory reaction controlled and directed by the immune system, in response to a trigger which might be relatively harmless to another individual. See also *immediate* and *delayed hypersensitivity* and *types I–IV hypersensitivity*.

Hypertrophy Enlargement of an organ due to an increase in the size of its cells. See also *hyperplasia*.

Hypovolaemia An abnormal decrease in blood volume in the circulation. See also *shock*.

Hypovolaemic shock A marked, possibly life-threatening, decrease in blood pressure due to decreased blood volume. Causes of hypovolaemic shock include severe *haemorrhage* or dehydration. Hypovolaemia would also occur where there has been major leakage of fluid from the circulation into the *interstitial fluid*. This might result when something causes a sudden increase in permeability (leakiness) of capillaries; this mechanism is part of the shock associated with some fatal infections. See also *shock, anaphylactic shock, cardiogenic shock, neurogenic shock, toxic shock* and *septic shock*.

Iatrogenic A disease or disorder directly caused by medical or surgical intervention.

Icterus The yellow discolouration of tissues caused by bile pigment in the circulation. Also called *jaundice*.

Idiopathic A disease or condition for which we do not (yet) know the cause, though it may have recognisable development processes, lesions or clinical signs. See also *aetiology, iatrogenic, hereditary, genetic* and *congenital diseases/conditions*.

Immediate hypersensitivity Also known as type I hypersensitivity. See *allergy* and *anaphylaxis*.

Immune response The specific defensive response by the host to foreign antigen. This response involves various cells and proteins of the immune system. The immune response is usually beneficial, though in some conditions it may be harmful by being inappropriate or excessive; alternatively, the immune system does not respond sufficiently to protect the host. See also *immunoglobulins, immunology, antibodies, antigen, antigenicity* and *hypersensitivity*.

Immunity Resistance to a disease because the host is able to defend itself from foreign antigens and make an immune response. See also *immune response, immunoglobulins, immunology, antibodies, antigen* and *antigenicity*.

Immunocompromise Failure of the immune system to function adequately for various reasons. See also *immuneosuppression*.

Immunodeficiency A state in which the immune system fails to function adequately. Immunodeficient animals are prone to other diseases. Divided into *primary* and *secondary immunodeficiencies*.

Immunoglobulins A protein produced as part of the immune response. See also *antibodies* and *globulins*.

Immunology The study of the immune system.

Immunostaining Immunological tests may be done on blood *serum* (this is called *serology*) but some immunological tests can also be carried out on tissues mounted on microscope slides, and this is then known as *immunostaining*. All types of cells of the body have their own 'fingerprint' of substances (usually proteins) carried on their outer surfaces; in a healthy individual, the immune system recognises these and does not start to react against them. Sometimes we can use this property of cells to confirm the diagnosis, for instance, if a pathologist is having trouble identifying a particular skin tumour under the microscope immunostains for specific cell types can be applied to the tissue and can help to reveal the identity of the tumour.

Immunosuppression When the immune system is inhibited by drugs or other processes. Immunosuppressed animals are prone to other diseases.

Incisional biopsy When only a representative part of a pathological lesion (such as a tumour or ulcer) is removed, fixed and sent to the pathologist for examination. The pathologist's diagnosis may then indicate whether more of the lesion should be removed or whether it can be treated without further surgery. See also *excisional biopsy*.

Incubation period The period of time between exposure of the animal to an infectious organism and the first appearance of clinical signs of disease caused by the organism. Also called *latent period* or *latency*.

Infarction Death (necrosis) of an area of tissue as a result of *ischaemia*. See also *ischaemia* and *perfusion*.

Inflammation A sequence of blood vascular and cellular events which occur in response to a potentially harmful stimulus. Inflammation attempts to remove the stimulus and prepare the tissue for repair. In some cases inflammation may be excessive or inappropriate and can then itself be harmful. See also *acute* and *chronic inflammation*.

Initiation In tumour formation, the transformation of a cell by a carcinogenic agent. See also *carcinogen* and *carcinogenesis*.

Innate immune system The first line of the body's defences; composed of chemical mediators of *inflammation, plasma proteins* and cells able to *phagocytose*, such as *neutrophils* and *macrophages*, and a type of *lymphocyte* called a *natural killer cell*. Also known as the *natural* or *native* immune system. Sometimes natural barriers of the body, which act as physical barriers to invasion, are classified as part of the innate immune system.

Interstitial fluid The fluid that is in the tissue spaces between cells. This fluid leaks from capillaries and is drained back to the blood circulation by the lymphatic vessels. See also *lymph*.

Interstitium The tissue spaces between cells. See also *interstitial fluid*.

Intussusception   When a tubular structure (such as a segment of the intestine) 'telescopes' into an adjacent segment.

Invasion   In cancer pathology, this is a trait of malignant tumour cells which enables them to infiltrate surrounding tissues and blood and lymph vessels, and thereby to spread (by *metastasis*).

Irreversible cell damage/change   A type of cellular change which occurs in response to a harmful (or physiological) stimulus from which the cell cannot recover if the damaging stimulus is removed. The cell seems to pass a 'point of no return' and cannot revert to normal and usually does not survive. See also *cloudy swelling, cellular degeneration, reversible cell damage* and *necrosis*.

Ischaemia   Decreased blood flow to an area of tissue and therefore decreased supply of vital nutrients, especially oxygen, to that area. See also *infarction* and *perfusion*.

-itis   Used at the end of a word to denote inflammation in the particular tissue, such as dermatitis or enteritis (inflammation in the skin and intestine, respectively). See *pleurisy* for an exception.

Jaundice   The yellow discolouration of tissues caused by bile pigment in the circulation. Also called *icterus*.

Keratinisation   The production of the hard horny protein, keratin, by cells. For instance, may happen in areas of wear and tear, such as on the elbows of elderly dogs. (Note that normal skin has a relatively thin protective layer of keratin on its surface.)

Labile cells   Cells that are continually dividing to replace lost cells, such as cells in the skin or the surface of the intestine. See also *stable, permanent* and *stem* cells.

Large granular lymphocytes   A type of *lymphocyte* that acts as part of the *innate immune system* and is able to destroy certain abnormal cells such as tumour cells and cells infected with viruses. Also known as *natural killer cells*.

Latent period   Period between an animal being exposed to the cause of a disease and the first clinical signs of the disease. Also called latency or *incubation period*.

Lesion   An abnormality associated with injury or cell damage.

Leucocytes   General term for white blood cells.

Leukaemia   Proliferation of neoplastic white blood cells. The abnormal cells circulate in the blood.

Liquefactive necrosis   A form of cell death (necrosis) in which the cell contents become liquefied by powerful enzymes, which degrade the dead cells and extracellular components. This type of necrosis is characteristic of insults to the brain such as infarction or bacterial infection. See also *necrosis, caseation necrosis, coagulative necrosis, fat necrosis, gangrene, wet gangrene, dry gangrene, moist gangrene* and *gas gangrene*.

Lymph   Clear fluid that flows within the lymphatic circulation.

Lymphadenopathy A non-specific term used to denote enlargement of the lymph nodes due to any cause.

Lymphocytes A small round white cell with a single nucleus. Lymphocytes are important in the immune response but they can also direct inflammatory responses. See also *memory cells.*

Lysosomes Vesicles in the cytoplasm of phagocytic cells that contain powerful protein-digesting enzymes. See also *phagocytosis.*

Macrophages Large phagocytic cells with single round nuclei. They are very efficient digesters of foreign material and do not necessarily die during the process (compare *neutrophils*). Macrophages are especially associated with chronic inflammation. See also *granulomatous inflammation, granuloma* and *phagocytosis.*

Malignant tumour A tumour whose cells are able to invade adjacent tissue and to spread, usually by lymph or blood vessels, to form secondary tumours (metastases) elsewhere in the body. See also *benign tumour, metastasis* and *neoplasia.*

Margination In acute inflammation, when white cells gather on the endothelial walls of small blood vessels in readiness for leaving the vessel and travelling to the site of inflammation. See also *acute inflammation.*

Mast cells Large round cells that are widespread in the body, tending to be positioned beside capillary beds. Mast cells produce potent chemicals which they store in granules in their cytoplasm. When they are stimulated (by a number of stimuli), the mast cells degranulate, releasing the chemicals. The contents of mast cell granules include *histamine*, which has several biological actions such as dilation, and increasing the leakiness, of blood vessels. See also *acute inflammation* and *type I hypersensitivity.*

Melaena Partially digested blood, from, for instance, a stomach ulcer, which gives the faeces a dark colour.

Memory cells *Lymphocytes* which are formed once an animal has been exposed to an *antigen*. These cells have the ability to mount a greater immune response compared to lymphocytes which have not previously encountered the antigen. See also *antigen* and *lymphocytes.*

Metaplasia Conversion of one mature tissue type into another. For instance alteration of an epithelium, like the lining of the urinary bladder, to a tougher more protective (squamous) one in response to *chronic inflammation*, in this case due to the presence of bladder stones, for example.

Metastasis The process in which cells from a malignant tumour invade adjacent tissue and spread, usually by lymph or blood vessels, to form secondary tumours (metastases) elsewhere in the body. See also *benign* and *malignant tumour* and *neoplasia.*

Metastatic calcification   Abnormal deposition of hard calcium in tissues when the level of calcium in the blood is abnormally high. See also *calcification* and *dystrophic calcification*.

Microbiology   A general term for the study of *infectious organisms*, more specifically, bacteriologists study bacteria, virologists study viruses, and mycologists study fungi and yeasts. Clinical samples, such as urine, pus, mucus or tissue may be sent to microbiology laboratories where potentially harmful infectious organisms associated with them can be grown in *culture* and identified. In the case of bacterial infection, the sensitivity of the organisms (i.e. which antibiotics may kill or limit its growth) can be assessed which gives the vet an indication of what treatment to use.

Mitosis   A form of cellular division in which the cell separates the chromosomes in its nucleus into two identical sets at the start of the process. Thus, the aim of mitosis in normal cells is that the two 'daughter' cells produced at the end are genetically identical to each other and to their parent cell.

Moist gangrene   A type of tissue death due to loss of blood supply. In this form of gangrene, pus-producing bacteria proliferate in the areas of necrosis. This type of gangrene characteristically appears rotten and is very foul smelling (putrefactive). See also *gangrene, dry gangrene, gas gangrene* and *wet gangrene*.

Monocytes   Immature macrophages circulating in the blood.

Multifactorial disease   A disease whose development and course is affected or modified by many factors and/or infectious agents. See also *aetiology* and *simple disease*.

Mutation   An alteration in the DNA of a cell, which may be the first stage in development of a tumour.

Native immune system   The first line of the body's defences. Also known as the *innate* or *natural* immune system. Sometimes natural barriers of the body (physical barriers to invasion) are classified as part of the innate immune system. See *innate immune system*.

Natural immune system   The first line of the body's defences. Also known as the *innate* or *native* immune system. See *innate immune system*.

Natural killer cells   A type of *lymphocyte* that acts as part of the *innate immune system* and is able to destroy certain abnormal cells such as tumour cells and cells infected with viruses. Also known as *large granular lymphocytes*.

Necropsy   Post-mortem dissections of animals involving examination of organs (called autopsies in human pathology). Usually, a report is written to describe the findings and may include the histopathological results as well. See *histopathology*.

Necrosis   Death of cells in a living organism, without specific reference to its cause. See also *gangrene, dry gangrene, gas gangrene, moist gangrene, wet gangrene, caseation, coagulative, liquefaction necrosis* and *fat necrosis*. Finally, compare with *autolysis*.

Neoplasia   The process by uncontrolled cell division leading to development of a neoplasm or tumour. Distinct from *hyperplasia*. See also *neoplasm* or *tumour*.

Neoplasm   A mass formed from abnormal and uncoordinated division of cells. The terms tumour or growth are also used. See also *tumour*.

Neurogenic shock   Dramatic decrease in blood pressure which may occur in animals when severely frightened or traumatised, or in extreme pain. Nerves stimulate dilation of blood vessels and so there is marked pooling of blood. Neurogenic shock may compound the effects of psychological shock (fright or trauma). See also *shock, anaphylactic shock, cardiogenic shock, hypovolaemic shock, toxic shock* and *septic shock*.

Neutropenia   A decrease in the number of circulating neutrophils in the blood. See also *leucopenia* and *pancytopenia*.

Neutrophil   A small phagocytic cell with a complex segmented nucleus (similar to an *eosinophil*; not a single round nucleus as in a *macrophage*). Neutrophils usually die in the process of *phagocytosis*. They are particularly associated with acute inflammation and with bacterial infections. See also *neutropenia*.

Neutrophilia   High numbers of neutrophils in the blood. Usually indicates a bacterial infection or acute inflammatory process in the body. See also *neutrophil* and *neutropenia*.

Nodular   Composed of small lumps or bumps (nodules) which are formed by proliferation or grouping of similar cells. Dense clusters of inflammatory cells may gather in the skin in certain skin conditions and the resulting swellings (nodules) can be palpated, or even seen in short-coated animals.

Noxious   Harmful or injurious. A noxious stimulus is something that causes cell or tissue damage.

Oedema   Abnormal accumulation of fluid in the tissues due to leakage from blood vessels or decreased drainage of lymph, or when there is general circulatory failure. Leakage from vessels occurs in acute inflammation or when vessel walls are damaged. Decreased drainage of lymph occurs when there is a tumour or fibrous scar blocking the lymph vessels. General circulatory failure occurs with severe heart disease.

-oma   Used at the end of a word, usually to denote a benign tumour, e.g. lipoma and hepatoma, as opposed to liposarcoma and hepatocarcinoma the malignant counterparts of these tumours. (Though note also melan*oma* and lymph*oma* are usually malignancies, and granul*oma*, which is a chronic inflammatory condition and not a neoplasm at all.)

Oncogenesis   The process by which neoplasms develop. See also *carcinogenesis* and *neoplasia* which are usually used interchangeably with oncogenesis.

-opathy   Used at the end of a word, usually to denote a pathological state or condition without being too specific as to type of process involved. Examples include lymphadenopathy, hepatopathy or dermatopathy being a pathological condition of the lymph glands, liver and skin, respectively, without reference to type of abnormality.

Organisation   The process of tissue repair by formation of spongy immature fibrous tissue with many capillaries (see *granulation tissue*) which is subsequently replaced by firmer collagenous fibrous tissue (see *fibrosis* or *scar tissue*). See also *tissue repair*.

Osmotic pressure   The pressure that develops due to differences in the concentration of solutes in water across a slightly leaky membrane (such as a capillary wall). In the body, solutes which exert osmotic pressure include *salts* and, especially important in the blood, *plasma proteins*.

Oxygen free radicals   Highly reactive forms of oxygen, which are products of metabolism, but which are normally removed by cellular processes. Under certain circumstances (exposure to ultraviolet light, or other radiation, for instance) the free radicals can build up in cells and be highly damaging to cellular structures.

Pancytopenia   A decrease in all cell types in the blood (white and red blood cells and *platelets*).

Paraneoplastic effect/syndrome   A disorder that develops in an animal with a neoplasm, which is indirectly linked to the tumour. An example of a paraneoplastic effect is the development of high blood calcium (hypercalcaemia) in an animal with lymphoma. This is due to the tumour secreting a substance that stimulates bone destruction, and the calcium level in the blood increases as a result of this bone destruction.

Parasite   An organism that lives on or in the body of the host, and which depends on the host for nutrition or protection or the correct environment for a certain stage (or stages) of its life cycle.

Passive immunity   The process by which young animals gain *immunity* from their mothers, by transfer of maternal *antibodies* during their time in the womb or by the consumption of colostrum soon after birth. Passive immunity is especially important for protection of the young from *pathogens* in their environment before they are able to mount an effective immune response themselves.

Pathogen   A non-specific term used to denote an infectious agent (e.g. bacteria, virus or fungus) capable of causing disease. See also *aetiology, aetiological agent, pathogenic factor* and *pathogenesis.*

Pathogenesis   Used when discussing how factors lead to disease, or the mechanisms of *disease development.* It describes the chain of events from the initial stimulus to the manifestation of the disease or the lesion produced.

Pathogenic factor   A factor that is capable of producing disease. An infectious agent capable of causing disease may often be referred to in non-specific terms as a *pathogen.* See also *aetiology, aetiological agent* and *pathogenesis.*

Pathognomonic   A pathological lesion or clinical sign which is absolutely characteristic or typical for a particular disease or condition.

Pathology   The study of the effects of disease on the body includes any deviation from a healthy or normal state in any living creature. Pathology encompasses a number of sub-divisions such as *general pathology, systematic* (or *special*) *pathology* and *clinical* (or *chemical*) *pathology.*

Pedunculated   On a stalk. Usually used to describe the appearance of tumours growing on stalks from body surfaces such as the skin.

Perfusion   The adequate circulation of blood to an area or tissue. See also *ischaemia* and *infarction.*

Permanent cells   Cells with limited, or no, capacity to divide and proliferate; they tend to last a long time and are not replaced when they die, e.g. brain cells. See also *stable cells* and *labile cells.*

Petechiae   Small discrete haemorrhages in the skin or within (or on) organs; smaller than *ecchymoses.* See also *haemorrhage* and *haematoma.*

Phagocytosis   The process by which certain cells engulf and digest a microbe, a foreign particle or another cell. See also *neutrophils* and *macrophages.*

Pinch biopsy   This is usually a small sample of tissue from an organ like the gut, upper respiratory tract or urogenital tract. A pinch biopsy is collected by taking a little chunk of the tissue using special forceps with an endoscope.

Plasma   The clear fluid portion of blood that remains after red and white cells and platelets are removed (usually the cells are made to sink to the bottom of the blood sample by spinning the blood very fast in a centrifuge). Plasma consists of water, salts, enzymes, *antibodies* and other proteins. It differs from *serum* in that plasma contains fibrinogen and other soluble clotting elements. See *plasma proteins.*

Plasma cells   A form of *lymphocyte* capable of producing *antibodies* as a part of the *humoral immune response.* Plasma cells are not really anything to do with plasma, other than the fact that antibodies they produce are included amongst the *plasma proteins*.

Plasma proteins   Proteins in blood that perform a variety of roles, including blood clotting, fighting diseases (*antibodies*), maintaining *osmotic pressure* and other important critical functions. They may also be referred to as serum proteins. See also *plasma*.

Platelets   Also called thrombocytes. Small cells circulating in the blood that are involved in blood clotting (haemostasis). During clotting, platelets clump together (aggregate) and adhere to the inner (*endothelial*) surface of a damaged vessel wall. Aggregation and adhesion of platelets along with the protein *fibrin* form the platelet plug part of a blood clot. Platelets do not have a nucleus.

Pleurisy   Inflammation of the pleura, the covering of the lungs. Tends to be used rather than the term pleuritis. See also *-itis*.

Pneumonia   Usually used to denote inflammation of the lungs. In fact, *pneumonitis* is the general term for inflammation of the lungs, whilst pneumonia is a type of pneumonitis specifically caused by infection. See also *-itis*.

Primary immunodeficiency   Disorder in which the immune system fails to function adequately due to an inherited defect in the immune system. See also *immunodeficiency* and *secondary immunodeficiency*.

Prognosis   The predicted progress of a disease and likelihood of recovery or length of survival of a patient after a particular diagnosis has been made. Knowing the prognosis for a disease helps determine which treatments to use. In veterinary medicine, knowing that a condition has a very poor prognosis can help us to make decisions on whether to try certain treatments, or to use supportive therapies, or even to put the animal to sleep to limit suffering.

Pruritus   Itchiness. Pruritus may predispose to *self-trauma* in many of our veterinary species. Note the spelling, with *-us* at the end and not *-is*; it is *not* an *-itis* word.

Punch biopsy   This is usually a small sample of tissue from an organ like the skin. Punch biopsies are collected by cutting a little core of the tissue using a special circular tool, a bit like a miniature cookie cutter.

Purulent   Contains *pus*. Related word is *purulence*. See also *pyo-* and *suppuration* or *suppurative*.

Pus   Creamy material containing live and dead *neutrophils*, necrotic tissue and bacteria. Note the spelling; one -s at the end and not two! Avoid use of the term pus-sy to describe something which contains pus, better to say pus-filled or *purulent* or *suppurative*. See also *abscess* and *suppuration*.

Pyo-   Used to denote pus production or suppuration, as in pyometra which is pus in the uterus. A pyogenic infection is one caused by types of bacteria that characteristically cause suppurative lesions. See also *purulent*.

Quiescent   May refer to cells that are 'resting', i.e. not dividing. Also used to mean cells that normally have a low level of division or proliferation (see *stable cells*).

Reactive   Used to denote something that happens in response to a stimulus. For instance, if an animal has an infected skin wound there may be a reactive increase in number (*hyperplasia*) of cells of the immune system (*lymphocytes*) in lymph nodes near to the wound. As a result of the lymphocyte hyperplasia the lymph nodes would increase in size – and this would also be considered a reactive change (reactive lymphaden*opathy*).

Recanalisation   One of the better consequences of *thrombus* formation. Small channels form through the thrombus and become lined by *endothelial* cells and therefore re-establish some blood flow through the previously blocked (thrombosed) vessel.

Regeneration   When a lesion heals with cells that are identical to the damaged and lost cells (i.e. as opposed to repair by *organisation*).

Repair   When damaged tissue heals, either by replacement of the lost cells by identical ones (*regeneration*) or by *organisation* (and *fibrosis*).

Retroviruses   Viruses that, amongst other effects on the host, are associated with causing certain neoplasms, e.g. feline leukaemia virus (FeLV) is a retrovirus implicated in formation of some tumours in cats.

Reversible cell damage/change   A type of cellular change which occurs in response to a harmful (or physiological) stimulus from which the cell can recover if the damaging stimulus is removed. See also *cloudy swelling*, *cellular degeneration*, *irreversible cell damage* and *necrosis*.

Sarcoma   A malignant tumour (neoplasm) originating from cells of connective tissue, or blood or lymphoid cells rather than cells of body surfaces. See also *carcinoma*.

Scar/scar tissue   Irreversible production of firm *collagenous* fibrous tissue in an area of marked or chronic damage. The collagen fibres in mature scars often contracts so that older scars appear puckered. See also *fibrosis* and *organisation*.

Sclerosis   Irreversible formation of large amounts of firm (*collagen*-containing or *collagenous*) fibrous tissue in an organ, usually due to chronic disease or damage. The affected organ feels tough and may be irregular if the fibrous tissue has contracted (like a *scar*) or if it is interspersed by little islands (nodules) of normal cells. Sclerosis of the liver in long-standing liver disease (or in chronic alcoholism) can cause the liver to become firm, shrunken and irregular (*nodular*).

Secondary immunodeficiency   Disorder in which the immune system fails to function adequately because another disease, disorder or condition in the body adversely affects the function of the immune system. See also *immunocompromise, immunodeficiency* and *primary immunodeficiency*.

Self-trauma   When animals damage themselves. Many skin conditions in our veterinary patients are altered or exacerbated by the animals scratching, licking or biting the area due to itchiness (*pruritus*) or due to altered or even loss of sensation. Self-trauma may also be a manifestation of a behavioural or stress-related problem, e.g. feather pecking in birds.

Septic   Infected. See also *septic shock, pus, abscess* and *suppuration*.

Septicaemia   A life-threatening condition which occurs when *pathogenic* bacteria are present and proliferating within the blood, causing *systemic* illness. See also *bacteraemia*.

Septic shock   Life-threatening decrease in blood pressure due to dilation of capillaries in the abdominal organs. A type of toxic shock, the toxins involved being bacterial toxins. See also *shock, anaphylactic shock, cardiogenic shock, hypovolaemic shock, neurogenic shock* and *toxic shock*.

Sequela(e)   A sequela is a pathological condition which results from another disease or injury. The plural is sequelae. An example of a sequela would be *ischaemic necrosis* in an organ as a result of blockage of a blood vessel by a *thromboembolus*. The sequelae of severe acute inflammation would include *ulceration, fibrosis* (scarring) and *abscessation*.

Serology   Use of blood *serum* to carry out immunological tests for diagnosis of diseases. Usually used for diagnosis of diseases caused by infectious organisms, in which specific *antibodies* produced by the immune system to the infectious agent can be detected, indicating that the animal has been exposed to the organism in question.

Serum   The clear fluid left behind when blood clots. It differs from *plasma* in that it does not contain *fibrinogen* nor many other soluble clotting factors (since these help to form the clot and therefore are removed from the liquid part of the blood when the clot forms).

Shock   A marked fall in blood pressure which is potentially life-threatening. In shock there is a mismatch between the total blood volume and the volume ('size') of the circulatory system (the blood volume is 'too small' to fill the circulatory system). Causes of shock include a decrease in the blood volume (*haemorrhage* or dehydration) or an effective decrease in the size of the circulatory system (by vasodilation) or acute failure of the heart to pump blood around the circulatory system. See also *anaphylactic shock, hypovolaemic shock, neurogenic shock, toxic shock* and *septic shock.*

Simple disease   A disease which has an uncomplicated development that could be summarised as aetiological agent + tissue = disease. See also *aetiology* and *multifactorial disease.*

Special pathology   The study of disease or disorder with reference to organ systems. Also called *systematic pathology.*

Specific immune system/response   Specific defence mechanisms in the body against infectious agents and other foreign molecules. See *adaptive immune system/response.*

Stable cells   Cells with long life spans which do not normally divide and proliferate but which can do so if required to (i.e. to replace lost cells or due to physiological needs which might stimulate *hyperplasia*). Examples of stable cells are epithelial cells in liver, kidney and lung. See also *permanent* and *labile cells.*

Stem cell   An 'immature' cell that can develop into a mature cell of any of a number of different cell types. So when a stem cell divides, each new cell has the potential to either remain as a stem cell or to become another type of cell with a more specialised function such as a muscle cell, a liver cell, or a brain cell.

Suppuration   Formation of *pus* as a sequela of acute inflammation. See also *abscess* and *pus.*

Suppurative   Used to describe something characterised by *pus* formation or *suppuration*, e.g. a suppurative skin wound. See also *purulence.*

Syndrome   A group of clinical signs and/or lesions that together is characteristic of a particular disease or disorder.

Systematic pathology   The study of the effects of disease with special reference to a specific tissue or a body system. For instance, dermatitis (inflammation in the skin) or osteosarcoma (neoplasia of bone) are examples of systematic or special pathological changes. Also known as *special pathology*. See also *general pathology* for contrast.

Systemic   Concerning all body systems, organs or tissues.

Thromboembolism   When a clot of blood travels from the site at which it formed in the blood circulation of a living animal and lodges, causing *ischaemia*. See also *thrombosis, thrombus* and *thromboembolus.*

Thromboembolus   A clot of blood that breaks away from a primary clot (*thrombus*) which has formed in the circulation of a living animal. The second clot, the thromboembolus, travels in the blood until it lodges somewhere else and can then produce *ischaemia*. See also *thrombosis, thrombus* and *thromboembolus.*

Thrombosis Blockage of blood vessels by a blood clot that forms within the circulatory system of a living animal. See also *thrombus, thromboembolus* and *thromboembolism*.

Thrombus A mass of coagulated blood, which forms within the circulatory system of a living animal. A thrombus may form at sites of *endothelial* damage or turbulent blood flow or when blood is especially thick (*Virchow's triad*). The plural is thrombi. See also *coagulation, disseminated intravascular coagulation* and *haemorrhage*.

Tissue regeneration When a lesion heals with cells that are identical to the damaged and lost cells (i.e. as opposed to repair by *organisation*).

Tissue repair When damaged tissue heals, either by replacement of the lost cells by identical ones (*regeneration*) or by *organisation* (and *fibrosis*).

Torsion When an organ or tissue twists around itself (such as a segment of intestine) or at its site of attachment or suspension (for instance, when the part of the peritoneum that suspends the spleen in the abdomen twists). Torsion can cause obstruction of a hollow organ, like the gut or uterus, but also compresses blood vessels running to the affected area and therefore can cause *ischaemia* and *oedema* of the tissue. See also *volvulus*.

Toxaemia Presence of a toxin in the blood circulation.

Toxicology In some cases, toxicologists may be asked to analyse samples for toxins or poisons, for instance, you or the pathologist might send stomach contents, urine or even fresh tissue from a necropsy of an animal suspected of having been poisoned.

Toxic shock Life-threatening decrease in blood pressure due to dilation of capillaries in the abdominal organs. The toxins involved being bacterial toxins. See also *shock, anaphylactic shock, cardiogenic shock, hypovolaemic shock, neurogenic shock* and *septic shock*.

Toxin A naturally produced substance which has a harmful effect; examples include venom produced by snakes or stinging insects, or poisons in certain plants, or harmful substances produced by some bacteria.

Transformation The process by which normal cells change to become neoplastic. See also *carcinogenesis, oncogenesis* or *neoplasia*.

Transudate The accumulation in tissues of fluid which has low protein content and which has leaked from the circulation due to low osmotic pressure in the blood or high blood pressure. See also *exudate* and *oedema*.

Tumour Strictly speaking, any swelling in the body, though is usually used to denote a neoplasm.

Tumour markers   Biological substances that are secreted by tumour cells and released into the blood (or other fluids). Tumour markers can be detected in samples of blood/fluid and can then aid diagnosis and *prognosis*.

Type I hypersensitivity reaction   Also known as immediate hypersensitivity. *Antigens* (or *allergens*) to which the animal is sensitised cause specific *antibodies* (*immunoglobulins*) to stimulate *mast cells*, making them release the contents of their intracytoplasmic granules (degranulate). The effects of this are dilation of nearby blood vessels and seepage of oedema and serum proteins (*exudate*) and, later, influx of inflammatory cells. In the respiratory tract the smooth muscle lining the airways also constricts (as in asthma) and in the skin, nerve endings are stimulated so there is extreme itchiness (*pruritus*). The effects can sometimes be more widespread leading to generalised anaphylaxis. See also *allergy*, *mast cells* and *histamine*.

Type II hypersensitivity reaction   Also known as *cytotoxic hypersensitivity*. An immune response in which elements of the immune system are directed to kill cells of the body because the target cells have been inappropriately coated with *antibodies*.

Type III hypersensitivity reaction   Damage caused to tissue by the accumulation of clumps of *antigen--antibody–complement protein* reactions (called *antibody complexes*) when there has been excessive immune stimulation. Presence of the complexes initiates *inflammation* which leads to the tissue damage. See also *complement*.

Type IV hypersensitivity reaction   Also known as *delayed-type hypersensitivity*. An inflammatory response, principally initiated by the actions of T lymphocytes, which can take several hours (24–72 hours) to develop after the sensitised animal is exposed to the stimulus to which it is sensitive.

Ulcer   An area of damage to a covering layer in the body (or epithelial surface) which involves the entire depth of the epithelium, exposing the underlying tissue. For instance, an ulcer of the epidermis of the skin exposes the underlying dermis and leaves it vulnerable to secondary infection. An ulcer of the epithelium of the stomach exposes the underlying tissues of the wall and can result in *haemorrhage* from blood vessels in the wall, or even penetration through the wall into the abdominal cavity. Compare *erosion*.

Urticaria   A red, swollen and very itchy (*pruritic*) reaction in the skin due to a type I hypersensitivity response. Popularly known as hives or a rash.

Vasculitis   Inflammation of the wall of blood vessels.

Vasoconstriction   Narrowing of a blood vessel due to contraction (or spasm) of the smooth muscle within its wall.

Vasodilation   Increase in the diameter of a blood vessel due to relaxation of the smooth muscle within its wall.

Vector   Refers to an animal, often an insect, which can carry an infectious agent and pass it between hosts. Examples of vectors would be the midge, which carries the bluetongue virus between susceptible ruminants, the mosquito which transmits heartworm to dogs and cats in some countries, and the flea, which is implicated in the transfer of a number of different infectious agents.

Vesicle   A fluid-filled lesion (commonly known as a blister) which occurs on the skin or on mucous membranes, such as in the mouth. Vesicles are delicate and the top surface usually gets damaged or ruptures to leave behind an *erosion* or *ulcer*, depending how deep the vesicle extended within the epithelial surface.

Viraemia   Presence of virus within the blood circulatory system.

Virchow's triad   The predisposing factors needed for formation of a *thrombus* in the circulatory system of a living animal. These are:
- Changes in vessel wall(s) such as physical damage (trauma), chemical injury, infection and bacterial *endotoxic* damage.
- Changes in flow (slow or turbulent flow).
- Changes in blood constituents (increased tendency to clot, also called *hypercoagulability*). This happens in renal failure, diabetes mellitus, heart failure, severe trauma or burns, and widespread cancer, for instance.

Any one of these three factors can result in thrombus formation, though in many conditions more than one factor will be present at the same time. See also *thrombus*.

Virulence   The ability of an infectious organism to cause disease after infecting a host.

Volvulus   Usually referring to a twist in the mesenteric suspension of the intestine which effectively forms a pinched-off or isolated loop of bowel. Volvulus is a cause of blockage (obstruction) of the intestine, also it can cause ischaemia of the gut wall due to blood vessels becoming compressed in the twist and can be a life-threatening condition. See also *torsion*.

Wet gangrene   A type of tissue death due to loss of blood supply. In this form of gangrene, bacteria are present and there is inflammation of adjacent non-necrotic tissue. The area swells and oozes fluid. See also *gangrene, dry gangrene, moist gangrene* and *gas gangrene*.

Wheal   A focal area of oedema in the skin, such as occurs after light trauma or insect bite.

Answers to Test Yourself Questions

This section suggests suitable answers to the test yourself questions for each chapter. Sub-headings tell you which chapter each block of six questions refer to. These are *suggested* answers, and you may have written answers in a slightly different way, which may still be perfectly correct; the idea is not to be 'word-perfect' with my answer but to make sure you understand the topics of the question in the first place.

Also, you may feel that I have included more information in some of my answers than the question seemed to require. This was deliberate! I hope that this section will serve as a useful revision aid for you, and that by putting my answers in context (which often means adding a bit of extra information) will help you to learn and understand the subjects more fully. Please note that in a written exam situation it is very important to make sure you 'answer the question'; giving masses of extra information to your examiner, which he or she has not actually asked you for, costs valuable time and may not gain you any extra points in the end. In an exam, remember to note how many marks are to be awarded for each question and tailor your answer accordingly.

Test yourself questions on Chapter 1

1. Definition of 'pathology'.

   From the Greek words, pathos – used in terms of suffering from a disease, and -logy used to infer 'study of' or 'science of'.

   The branch of medical science that involves study of the causes of diseases, how they develop and their effects on the body. It encompasses any deviation from a healthy or normal condition in any living creature.

   The effects of diseases are studied at the level of the whole body, the organs or tissues, the cells and within cells (sub-cellular level).

2. The work of (a) anatomic pathologists and (b) clinical pathologists:

   a. Anatomic pathologists study disease by looking at tissue and organs, such as in post-mortem examinations (*necropsies*), or by looking at tissues from live animals (called *biopsies*).

      Anatomic pathologists look at the tissues/organs by eye (gross examination) to identify abnormalities and under the microscope (histology slides).

   b. Clinical pathologists assess disease by studying body fluids (e.g. blood, urine, joint fluid, abdominal tap fluid, cerebrospinal fluid etc.).

      They may look at the chemical composition (*clinical biochemistry*) or use a microscope to study a stained smear of the sample on a glass microscope slide to examine the types of cells in the fluid or in a fine-needle aspirate (FNA) (called *cytology*).

Clinical pathologists might also see bacteria or other infectious organisms in a cytology preparation.

Haematology is specifically the study of cell types in blood.

3. a. Organisms studied by microbiologists.

Microbiologists study infectious organisms such as bacteria, viruses, fungi and yeasts.

b. Still thinking about microbiology, what is meant by 'sensitivity' and why is it helpful and/or important?

Clinical samples may be sent to microbiology laboratories where they can grow (*culture*) and identify bacteria. *Sensitivity* means identifying which antibiotics the organism is likely to be killed by. This is important because it gives the vet an indication of what antibiotic treatment to use, and (for a bonus mark!) may help to reduce the development of resistance to antibiotics by bacteria.

4. Some sensible actions to take if involved in a case which involves the police or other authorities:

i. Seek advice (pathology laboratory, veterinary forensic pathologist, University Pathology Department) unless experienced in dealing with such cases.

ii. Keep careful notes, photographs, logged telephone calls or case records securely and safely stored.

iii. Any biological material, including bodies of deceased animals, should be logged and labelled, and stored securely until removal by an authorised person.

5. Why are veterinary pathologists important for the health of human beings?

Veterinary pathologists involved in maintaining herd- or flock-health on farms and nationally help to prevent widespread infectious diseases and to protect food quality and safety.

Veterinary pathologists may also be the first to recognise 'zoonotic' diseases – these are diseases able to pass from animals to man.

6. 'General' pathology and 'systemic' or 'special' pathology:

i. General pathology is the study of processes in disease and is not necessarily limited to discussion of a particular tissue or organ.

ii. Systematic (special) pathology is the study of the effects of disease with reference to a specific tissue or body system.

Test yourself questions on Chapter 2

1. Definition of 'aetiology' (or etiology).

Aetiology means the study or science of the causes of disease.

2. What does it mean if a factor is described as 'pathogenic'?
    The factor is capable of producing disease.
    Also, an infectious agent (bacteria, virus and fungus) capable of causing disease may often be referred to in non-specific terms as a *pathogen*.
3. Classification of aetiological agents, including examples.

An example of classification of aetiological agents – you may prefer to use a different classification system

Internal factors

- Genetic – *defects* or *mutations*

- Immune system – *defects* or *abnormal responses*

- Aging – *natural* processes or *premature* aging

External factors

- Physical – *trauma, pressure* etc.

- Chemical – *toxins, poisons, heavy metals* etc.

- Infectious – *parasites, bacteria, viruses, fungi* etc.

- Environmental – *nutrition (deficiencies or excesses)*

    – temperature

    – hygiene

    – radiation, e.g. ultraviolet light

---

4. Short notes on the differences between (i) acquired diseases, (ii) congenital diseases and (iii) idiopathic diseases:
    i.   *Acquired diseases* develop at some stage during life as a result of the effects of one or more aetiological agent acting during life.
    ii. *Congenital diseases* are diseases which the animal is born with. Congenital diseases occur because the aetiological agent acts on the embryo or foetus, on the uterus or placenta, or on the mother, either before or during pregnancy. Clinical signs of a congenital disease are not necessarily seen at birth, but may show up later in life.
    iii. *Idiopathic diseases* are diseases of which we do not (yet) know the cause, though they may have recognisable development processes, lesions or clinical signs.

5. Suggest up to six factors which may modify the course of a multi-factorial disease in an animal, including those factors which make disease more likely to occur in a particular animal.

    Housing in groups, over-crowding, age (very old or very young), breed, species, other diseases or infections, some drugs, not vaccinated or no immunity, no colostrum (first milk) from the mother, inappropriate immune response (too little or too much), nutritional state (hunger, malnutrition or obesity), genes, thirst, poor hygiene in the environment, poor air-quality, fatigue, inappropriate or poor husbandry, 'stress', . . . you may be able to think of more factors.

Test yourself questions on Chapter 3

1. Short notes to define 'lesion':
    i. Structural and functional changes.
    ii. *Pathological changes* in tissues or organs. Both gross changes – abnormalities we can see, and changes *in the cells* which make up that tissue or organ (*cellular changes*).
    iii. These changes occur in response to *injurious* or harmful *stimuli* (*aetiological agents*).
    iv. *Reversible cell injuries* (the harmful stimulus causes alteration or loss of cell function and structural changes but the cell recovers if the stimulus is removed) or *irreversible cell injuries* (cell injury causes alteration or loss of cell function and structural changes, but the cell *cannot* recover if stimulus stops or is removed, i.e. cell dies).
    v. Examples of reversible injuries are *cell adaptations* such as *some changes in cell growth,* and *cellular degeneration.* Examples of irreversible cell injuries are *neoplastic transformation* and *necrosis.*

2. Examples of cellular degeneration and associated clinical signs or conditions.

    Note that you may have found other examples of clinical signs or conditions associated with cellular degeneration during your reading of clinical experience; these are just some examples:
    i. Accumulation of *cellular components* in aging cells.
    ii. *Hydropic change* (fluid swelling), e.g. liver cell damage by toxins.
    iii. *Fatty change* – fat accumulating in cells because of increased or long-term fat breakdown in the body, e.g. malnutrition, decreased metabolism of cells damaged by toxins, or reduced oxygen supply due to heart dysfunction.
    Note also idiopathic fatty change in the livers of older cats.

iv. *Pigments*, e.g. endogenous – includes haemosiderin (after haemorrhage), bile (in jaundice), melanin (in chronic dermatitis); exogenous – includes carbon (from pollution), tattoo inks.

v. *Proteins*, e.g. *viral inclusions*.

3. Coagulative necrosis:

i. The most common form of necrosis, occurring in many of the 'solid' organs.

ii. Organs retain their structure but are pale and firm as though cooked.

iii. The dead cells often retain their outline when viewed under the microscope but are pale-staining and ghost-like. Inflammatory cells move in to start to remove the dead cells (demolition phase of healing).

iv. Proteins are released into the blood by the damaged and dying cells and are useful diagnostically, e.g. creatine kinase (CK) (indicate muscle damage) and alanine aminotransferase (AAT) (indicate liver damage).

4. Sequelae of necrosis (apart from tissue regeneration):
   ○ scar formation
   ○ ulceration
   ○ sequestration

5. a. *Calcification* is the deposition of calcium salts in *normal* or *abnormal* tissues and affected tissue is hard or gritty to touch and the calcium deposition can be felt as a scraping sensation when the tissue is incised with a knife.

   b. *Dystrophic calcification* is the deposition of calcium in areas of tissue damage (especially necrosis).

   c. *Metastatic calcification* is the deposition of calcium associated with *persistently high body calcium levels*, such as occurs in vitamin D toxicity, excess parathyroid hormone (or parathyroid-like hormone produced by certain tumours) and renal failure.

6. *Gout* occurs as articular, renal and visceral forms in birds, snakes and mink.

   Uric acid crystals and urates deposit in tissues when there is excess production or insufficient excretion of the metabolic waste-product uric acid. When uric acid levels in blood exceed a certain level, the uric acid crystallises from solution at various sites causing inflammation and pain.

Test yourself questions on Chapter 4

1. Definition of inflammation with brief notes:
   • A complex progression of blood vascular and tissue changes that develop in response to tissue injury.

- A primarily protective response which extends various defensive mechanisms of the blood (phagocytic cells, leucocytes and antibodies) out into the tissues.
- Prepares the way for repair of the tissue.
- Often works with, and is directed by, cells of the immune system.
- Under certain circumstances uncontrolled or inappropriate inflammation is harmful or destructive (even life-threatening if severe).
- In veterinary species, inflammation is often exacerbated by self-trauma – scratching, licking, biting etc. – which can cause further tissue damage or introduce infection.
- Described as acute or chronic which infers not just the duration but also indicates differences in the inflammatory cells involved.
- Usually indicated by the ending '-itis' after the Greek word for the organ, e.g. hepatitis, nephritis, enteritis, colitis, dermatitis etc.

2. a. The three phases of acute inflammation:
    - vascular
    - exudative
    - cellular
    b. The five (local) clinical (or cardinal) signs of acute inflammation and the phase(s) likely to contribute:
    - redness – vascular phase
    - heat in the tissue – vascular
    - pain – vascular and exudative phases, plus chemical messengers from inflammatory cells – i.e. cellular phase.
    - swelling – exudative (vascular)
    - loss of function – due to pain and swelling, so see two previous bullet points

3. a. Why is the tissue fluid which results in the exudative phase of acute inflammation high in protein?
        Capillaries are made leaky by the opening up of gaps between the endothelial cells, large molecules in the blood (like proteins) and cells are able to escape into the tissues. Normally, proteins and cells are too large to pass through the intercellular junctions in the capillary walls.
    b. Typical components of an inflammatory exudate.
        Water, electrolytes (salts), plasma proteins (albumin, globulin and fibrinogen), erythrocytes (red blood cells) and platelets.

4. Describe how an abscess may form.
    Suppurative exudate can become walled off by fibrous tissue and remain as a pocket of inflammation which refuses to clear up or occasionally bursts out.

5. Brief discussion of the difference between acute and chronic inflammation:

- Acute inflammation is the initial reaction of a tissue to injury which aims to rapidly contain, dilute and remove the harmful stimulus, and to prepare the tissues for repair. Acute inflammation involves the blood vascular system (vascular phase) and exudation of protein-rich fluid from the blood into the surrounding damaged tissue. Inflammatory cells, especially neutrophils, are recruited to the area and leave the blood circulation in the exuded fluid, and then to help to destroy the cause of the inflammation (phagocytosis). Mast cells are important as they contain granules which they release and which dilate blood vessels and make them leaky – allowing exudation and leucocyte recruitment.

- Chronic inflammation is the persistence of the inflammatory response for longer than approximately 10–14 days (perhaps up to year or more). Chronic inflammation is not exudative and involves the formation of fibrous tissue and different cells, such as macrophages, and cells of the immune system (lymphocytes and plasma cells). Mast cells and neutrophils play lesser roles in chronic inflammation, if they are involved at all. Chronic inflammation may also be accompanied by reactive hyperplasia or hypertrophy in surrounding tissues, as the mediators which encourage fibrous tissue formation can stimulate division and growth of other cells too.

6. a. The two main types of chronic inflammation and the appearance of each of these types of chronic inflammatory response.

Granulomatous and non-granulomatous (or diffuse) chronic inflammation, according to the pattern of inflammatory cells seen under the microscope.

Non-granulomatous chronic inflammation – tissue may thicken and may look and feel 'leathery'.

Granulomas may be single and large (forming a well-defined lump), or smaller and multiple – so tissue feels thickened and nodular ('knobbly' or containing lots of small lumps).

b. Simple diagram of a granuloma indicating arrangement of the main cell types involved (see Box 4.14).

Central macrophages and possibly neutrophils and multinucleated giant cells, with other mainly mononuclear inflammatory cells (lymphocytes and plasma cells) clustered around the macrophages and a rim of fibrous tissue around the outside.

c. Example of a disease characterised by granulomatous inflammation

Feline infectious peritonitis (FIP), tuberculosis, some parasitic diseases, some hypersensitivities and immune responses. I would allow feline eosinophilic granuloma!

You could have foreign body response to splinters or sutures too – things that resist destruction by the acute inflammatory response.

Test yourself questions on Chapter 5

1. List the first lines of defences of animals against invading infectious organisms:
   - Innate (natural or native) immunity – chemical mediators of inflammation, several plasma proteins, phagocytic cells, such as *neutrophils, macrophages* and *natural killer cells.*
   - Adaptive (*acquired* or *specific*) immunity.
   - Natural barriers of the body including the epithelial covering surfaces of structures such as the skin, respiratory or urinary tracts or gut.
   - In some areas, epithelial surfaces are further protected by mucus, fats (e.g. sebum) or protein, or by the cilia.
2. '*Antigen*' is formed from the words antibody generating.
3. True/false questions
   - i. True.
   - ii. False: Whilst they are *especially* associated with organs of the lymphoid system (lymph nodes and lymph, bone marrow, spleen and the thymus in young animals), lymphocytes are found throughout the body tissues and in the blood.
   - iii. True: Lymphocytic cells belong to the B cell line or the T cell line; each line has different specific roles in the immune response.
   - iv. False: A major role of plasma cells is to manufacture large quantities of antibodies, and not to phagocytose bacteria.
   - v. True.
   - vi. False: Antibodies are formed from paired chains of proteins in a 'Y' shape but it is the variable region at the tips of the 'Y' shape which gives the antibody its specificity to a particular antigen, and not the bonds joining the chains.
   - vii. True: Specific antibody-producing B cells have 'memory', and will respond more quickly and to a greater extent in vaccinated animals.
   - viii. False: Antibodies themselves cannot kill invading microorganisms; they simply 'label' the organism so that another part of the immune system can destroy it, e.g. the complement cascade.
   - ix. True: The antigen is 'presented' to the T helper cells by other cells called antigen-presenting cells – these include

macrophages, B cells and dendritic cells. If the T cell has the correct antigen receptor and 'recognises' the antigen as something foreign or harmful, it will respond by helping to initiate an immune response.

x. False: T cell responses also have 'memory', in fact specific T cells called *memory T cells* persist after an immune response to a particular antigen has subsided.

4. Some important conditions associated with immunodeficiency:
   - *Primary immunodeficiencies*, i.e. uncommon congenital disorders in animals, suspected when there are persistent or repeated bouts of infectious disease in young animals.
   - *Physiological states* such as age, breed, gender, pregnancy, season of the year, stress and trauma, diet and hormones.
   - *Chronic diseases*, especially certain viruses, which appear to interfere with function of cells, such as lymphocytes or neutrophils.
   - *Passive immunity* is the mechanism whereby young animals gain immunity from their mothers by transfer of the mother's antibodies during their time in the womb, or by the consumption of colostrum within 12–48 hours after birth.
   - *Failure of passive immunity* – animals that do not consume sufficient colostrum, perhaps because they are too weak to stand, or their mothers are too poorly to allow suckling, may be vulnerable to infections early in life.

5. a. Definition of 'hypersensitivity'
      Hypersensitivities (or hypersensitivity reactions) are excessive reactions mediated by the immune system to stimuli which would not be harmful in a normal animal.
   b. Notes on one type:
      - *Type I hypersensitivity (immediate hypersensitivity)*, the basis of acute *allergic responses*. Antigens (or allergens) to which the animal is sensitised cause specific *antibodies (immunoglobulins)* to stimulate mast cells to degranulate. This leads to dilation of nearby blood vessels and seepage of exudate and, later, influx of inflammatory cells to the area. Additional effects, depending on where the mast cell response occurs, include smooth muscle constriction in the respiratory tract and stimulation of nerve endings in the skin (causing pruritus). The mast cell degranulation can sometimes be more widespread leading to generalised anaphylaxis, which causes shock. Eosinophils may be present – attracted to degranulating mast cells. They may release the contents of their own granules causing tissue damage and secondary inflammation.
      - *Type II hypersensitivity (cytotoxic hypersensitivity)*. Elements of the immune system directed to kill cells of the body

because the target cells have been inappropriately labelled with antibodies as 'foreign' or 'harmful'.

- *Type III hypersensitivity.* Tissue damage caused by the accumulation of antigen, antibody and complement proteins which form antibody or immune complexes – clumps of antigen, antibody and complement proteins which would normally be destroyed by phagocytosis cells. When there has been excessive immune stimulation the complexes can build up and resist degradation. The immune complexes may remain at their site of formation or circulate in the blood stream and lodge elsewhere. They stimulate local inflammation which then causes damage to surrounding tissues, such as widespread vasculitis.
- *Type IV hypersensitivity (delayed-type hypersensitivity).* An inflammatory response involving cells of the immune system, which can take several hours to develop after the sensitised animal is exposed to the stimulus to which it is sensitive. Involves initially T helper cells, also macrophages and B lymphocytes, and later more macrophages, lymphocytes and neutrophils (via chemical messengers secreted by the initially stimulated immune cells).

6. a. Definition of autoimmunity.

   When the immune system mounts an immune response against the body's own tissues because normal proteins on the surface of cells are regarded as 'foreign'. Mechanisms, include failure of regulatory control of the immune system or new exposure of self-antigens that are normally in protected sites. Certain viruses may trigger autoimmunity by mimicking normal proteins, for instance!

   b. Treatment of autoimmune diseases and side effects.

   Treatment broadly involves controlling the inappropriate immune response by dampening down the immune system. This can have the unwanted effect of making the animal vulnerable to other diseases, especially infections.

Test yourself questions on Chapter 6

1. Extent to which the new tissue is the same as the tissue that was previously there depends on:
   - the *regenerative capacity* of the cells in tissue
   - the *extent* of the defect to be filled
2. Regeneration – replacement by cells of the same type since the surrounding living cells multiply and fill in the gap left by the dead

cells. To do this, the cells that make up the tissue must be able to divide by the process of *mitosis*.

Whereas organisation refers to replacement by fibrovascular connective tissue (scar tissue), which occurs when cells are not able to regenerate themselves, or where there has been a large area of necrosis so living regenerative cells are further away from the centre of the area of damage or cannot fill the gap quickly enough.

3. The three phases of organisation:
    *   *Demolition* or *inflammatory* phase. This is the phase in which 'cleaning-up' of the wound or damaged tissue occurs. This is performed mainly by neutrophils and macrophages, though lymphocytes, plasma cells and eosinophils may be involved under some circumstances.
    *   *Granulation* phase. In the granulation phase immature connective tissue (*granulation tissue*) is formed to start to fill in the wound.
    *   *Maturation* phase. In the maturation phase, the immature fibrous tissue formed in the phase of granulation matures by a process called fibrosis. The result of this phase is formation of a fibrous scar.
4. Healing where there has been epithelial damage only:
    *   When the epidermis is damaged there will be exudation of serum which will dry and form a scab of dried serum protein (fibrin), possibly with dead and dying white cells, such as neutrophils.
    *   Scab serves to protect the next stage which is proliferation of the epidermis from around the edge of the wound. The epithelial cells proliferate readily by mitosis since they are labile cells.
    *   The proliferating cells move across to form a continuous layer beneath scab. Eventually, the scab falls away revealing the newly regenerated and healed epidermis beneath. In this case there is minimal granulation tissue and fibrosis (scar formation).
5. Healing of a clean incised (surgical) wound versus larger, irregular, contaminated wound.

    The surface epidermis will regenerate as described in your answer to question 4. Underneath the epidermal layer a soft protein plug of fibrin will form. This will be replaced (in 5–7 days) by a slender seam of granulation tissue (by organisation) and by mature fibrosis (scar) in 2–3 weeks. This process is known as healing by primary union or first intention.

    Whereas if there is a tissue defect the edges of the wound are widely separated and the defect contains exudate and necrotic debris (and possibly bacteria). In this case the defect fills in by granulation, maturing to fibrosis, but more of it must form to fill the gap. As before the fibrous tissue matures, possibly taking several weeks, and the resulting scar will be larger than with first intention healing and may be less cosmetic. This process is known as healing by secondary union or second intention.

6. What can impair, prevent or alter healing?
   Choose from the following:
   - Severe prolonged damage with loss of the connective tissue framework or too many of the cells have been damaged to be able to regenerate the tissue (or they are permanent cells). These conditions tend to favour repair by fibrosis.
   - Contamination – exudate, dirt, bacteria and necrotic tissue.
   - Inadequate blood supply.
   - Systemic hormonal disorders – such as diabetes mellitus, hyper-adrenocorticism which alter metabolism and activity of cells.
   - Inadequate nutrition – protein and energy are particularly important for healing.
   - Movement, such as inadequate immobilisation of a healing limb, causes wound edges to move against each other.
   - Self-trauma – licking, biting, scratching of wounded areas, allowing bacterial contamination or irritation, and prolonging inflammation and slowing healing.
   - Old age – blood circulation may be poorer and state of nutrition more variable.
   - Immunodeficiency diseases – immune cells direct the inflammatory phase of organisation. Impaired immune function also allows bacterial contaminants to survive.
   - Chemotherapeutic drugs and radiation have detrimental effects on actively dividing cells, including the cells important in healing.
   - Denervation alters movement of limbs, decreases blood supply and may encourage self-trauma due to reduced pain sensation in the affected area.

Test yourself questions on Chapter 7

1. Answer to true/false questions.
   i. True: Capillaries are very small but very numerous, so their total volume means that all together they can contain a huge amount of blood – this is significant in development of shock.
   ii. False: Capillaries form fine networks, or capillary beds which are situated between the arterial flow (blood from the heart) and the venous flow (blood returning to the heart). The amount and speed of blood flow in these areas is affected by various influences.

iii. False: Capillary walls are not much more than a single-layered crazy paving of endothelial cells.

iv. False: Capillaries are normally slightly leaky, so there is a small net outflow of fluid from capillaries into surrounding tissues (known as interstitial fluid). Interstitial fluid bathes the cells and tissues but is 'outside' of the blood vessels.

v. False: Lymph vessels are thinner walled and are at lower pressure than most blood vessels.

vi. True: Like blood vessels lymph vessels are of various sizes, starting small (like capillaries) and getting gradually larger as they drain back towards the blood circulatory system somewhere near the right side of the heart.

vii. True: Lymph vessels have lymph nodes at intervals, which act as filters and are important in the function of the immune system.

viii. False: Oedema is the accumulation of interstitial fluid in the tissues which causes a soft swelling of the tissue, which can be 'pitted'. There are different types of oedema but in all of these types of oedema, the lymphatic circulation is not able to remove adequately the excess fluid from the tissues.

ix. True.

x. False: Though there are some situations in which oedema may be damaging and even life-threatening (oedema of the lungs, brain or larynx, for instance). In most instances, oedema is an indication of something else going wrong in the body (e.g. heart disease) but it may not necessarily be harmful in itself.

2. a. Contrast the terms *ischaemia* and *infarction*.

   Ischaemia is decreased blood flow or *perfusion* and therefore decreased supply of vital nutrients, especially oxygen, to an area. *Infarction* means death (necrosis) of the area of tissue as a result of ischaemia (i.e. an infarct is an area of ischaemic necrosis in a tissue or organ).

   b. Six common causes of ischaemia.

   You should have included thrombosis, vasoconstriction, embolism, compression, vasculitis and vessel damage. See Box 7.6 for diagrams (you could have included simple diagrams in your answer).

   c. Global infarction.

   Global infarction occurs when there is blockage of a large or proximal artery (artery nearer the heart) which is responsible for supplying blood to a wider area of tissue; in this case, there will be more severe or extensive infarction of the tissue than a focal infarction due to blockage of a smaller artery.

d. Simple flow diagram to illustrate the stages of development of an infarct. Something like this would do, though you may have your own version.

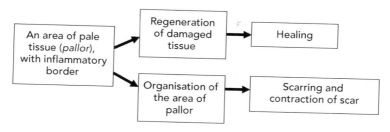

3. a. The part played by fibrinogen in blood coagulation.

Blood clotting depends to a large extent on conversion of fibrinogen in the blood to an insoluble form called fibrin. Strands of fibrin are part of the structure of a blood clot.

b. Why vitamin K is important to blood coagulation?

Formation of fibrin is brought about by a cascade of enzymes called clotting factors, produced by the liver. The inactive form of each factor is activated in sequence during the clotting cascade, each newly formed active factor then activates the next factor in the chain. Several steps in the cascade require vitamin K to help the reactions to occur.

4. a. Factors which determine the clinical significance of haemorrhage in animals:

* *Where the bleeding occurs* – e.g. haemorrhage into a low-pressure area, such as the abdomen will continue almost unchecked if not treated. Any clots formed may be simply 'pushed' off by the force of blood behind them. Whereas bleeding into an area which has higher local pressure, such as into a muscle in the case of a large bruise, is more likely to slow and possibly stop on its own.

* *How fast the bleeding occurs* – again relates to pressure in the surrounding area but also which type of vessel is bleeding. Arteries are at higher pressure than veins and will bleed faster than a vein and the blood loss will be more serious and less likely to clot without treatment. The speed of blood loss determines how sick the animal becomes since an animal can adapt to slow loss of blood, whereas rapid loss of blood will cause sudden serious decrease in blood pressure (shock).

* *How much blood is lost* – again, small slow losses can be compensated for by increased production of blood cells in the marrow and increased intake or retention of fluid. Large

losses exhaust the marrow and be more difficult for the animal to recover from.

b. A dog in your care develops black tarry faeces – what would you suspect was happening in the digestive tract, and where?

How about if there was fresh blood in the faeces?

Black and tarry faeces suggest bleeding into the digestive tract (or melaena). Furthermore, since it is black and tarry, you would suspect that the blood has been partially digested, which suggests the bleeding is in the 'higher' digestive tract (e.g. a bleeding gastric ulcer). Fresh blood would suggest lower tract bleeding – e.g. a haemorrhage in the large intestine (inflammation or tumour, for instance).

5. a. What is meant by embolus?

A mass of material able to lodge in a vessel and block it.

b. Brief description of thromboembolus in the case of heart valve diseases – an embolus derived from a thrombus, i.e. a bit of a larger intravascular blood clot that breaks away and travels in the circulation until it lodges in smaller vessels and blocks it.

In some heart diseases, thrombi form on the heart valves (Virchow's triad applies). Portions of these thrombi may break away and travel in the circulation. The resulting effects depend on which side of the heart the valvular thrombi originally formed.

- Valvular thrombosis on the left side of the heart can lead to emboli in the systemic circulation.
- Valvular thrombosis on the right side of the heart can lead to emboli in the pulmonary circulation (lungs).

c. Three examples of other forms of embolus.

Choose from:

- Embolus of *tumour cells.*
- *Parasitic* embolus, e.g. heartworm (*dirofilaria*) larvae in the lungs of affected dogs.
- *Fat* emboli, after the fracture of a long bone fractures.
- *Infective/inflammatory* emboli composed of infectious agents, necrotic tissue, leucocytes, fibrin circulating from a site of infection or inflammation; infection may be spread around the body this way (*haematogenous spread*).
- *Foreign* material may follow exposure of the circulatory system by injury, injection or surgery, when foreign material could potentially enter the bloodstream and travel to another site, could establish secondary granulomatous inflammation (*foreign body response*).
- *Fibrocartilage* emboli – when the cartilage and fibrous cushion of degenerate vertebral discs enter the blood stream and lodge somewhere.

- *Gas* emboli – gas or air bubbles can lodge in the bloodstream and act as solid obstructions.

6. a. Define 'shock'.

   A state of circulatory collapse, resulting in a severe state of reduced blood perfusion of tissue blood or a mismatch between the total blood volume, and the volume of the circulatory system.

   b. Brief outline of the main types of shock according to the way they develop.

   Hypovolaemic shock – shock due to decreased blood volume, e.g. severe haemorrhage or dehydration, sudden increased permeability ('leakiness') of capillaries, as in fatal infections.

   Vasodilation – marked increase in 'size' of the circulatory system in comparison to the amount of blood it holds, and therefore lack of effective circulation. Usually occurs in the very numerous capillaries, which have a huge potential volume, so when dilated the blood effectively 'pools' in the capillary beds.

   Cardiogenic shock – acute cardiac failure causes severe marked decrease in cardiac output because the heart is suddenly unable to pump the blood effectively.

   c. Five typical clinical signs of shock.
   Choose from:
   - Cold extremities
   - Core temperature high or low depending on cause of shock
   - Shivering in early stages
   - Heart rate may be increased or may be irregular and/or decreased
   - Weak peripheral pulse
   - Collapsed circulation (it may be hard to find a vein for intravenous injections or infusions)
   - Respiratory rate may be increased initially but may decrease if animal loses consciousness
   - Pale or discoloured (brick red or even blue) mucous membranes
   - Slow capillary refill times
   - Lethargy, lack of interest in surroundings, depression (and these effects may be accompanied or exacerbated by signs of pain, if shock is due to blood loss after trauma)
   - Loss of consciousness
   - Muscle weakness
   - Decreased urine production
   - Decreased blood pressure

You may have seen or read of other clinical signs of shock in addition to this list.

Test yourself questions on Chapter 8

1. a. List of four common reversible cell adaptations/changes involving altered cell growth or size:
   i. atrophy
   ii. hypertrophy
   iii. hyperplasia
   iv. metaplasia
   b. A simple diagram to illustrate the changes in part 1.a.
      You could have got quite creative here or done something really simple like this diagram:

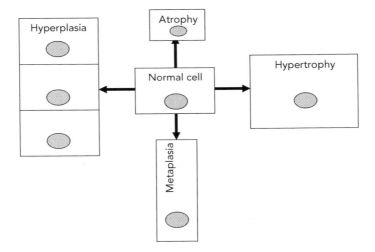

   c. Define neoplasia and indicate what fundamental way neoplasia differs from the changes listed in part 1.a.
      The key point is that neoplasia is a non-reversible change and neoplastic cells cannot revert to normal once the stimulus is removed. This is unlike atrophy, hypertrophy, hyperplasia and metaplasia, which are reversible.
      You could also have noted that normal cells communicate with each other and usually grow in a coordinated manner, stopping division when no more cells are required. Neoplastic cells, on the other hand, lack this coordination with normal tissue and go on growing and dividing in an uncontrolled manner.
      You could possibly have noted also that the neoplastic cell loses its normal differentiation.

2. a. Stages of changes to the genetic make-up of a cell fundamental to tumour development.
   - Initiation – a trigger factor or event that causes irreversible changes to the genes of a cell (transforming the cell)
   - Promotion – a factor or event that causes the transformed cell to proliferate (forming a tumour)
   - Progression – spontaneous occurrence of new changes to the genes of the offspring of the transformed cell, which may increase the malignant behaviour of the tumour

   b. List of groups of carcinogenic factors for domestic animals.

   You may have decided to be more specific and name particular chemicals, or various types of radiation (like ultraviolet or radioactive radiation), but I have opted to be more general. However, you answer it, in an exam situation you need to be sure to include only substances which are scientifically proven to be associated with cancer development.
   - chemicals
   - viruses
   - radiation
   - hormones
   - bacteria
   - parasites

3. Simple table outlining common differences between benign and malignant tumours.

   Something along the lines of the following table would do:

Benign tumours	Malignant tumours
Tumour more likely to be slow-growing	Tumour more likely to be rapidly growing (aggressive)
Tumour discrete – can be relatively easily identified and 'shelled-out' at surgery	Tumour may have an irregular outline; hard to identify edges of tumour at surgery
No indication of invasion of adjacent tissue seen histologically	Invasion of adjacent tissues and/or vessels
Tumour may have a capsule around it Do not metastasise Necrosis unlikely Cells and nuclei are relatively uniform Cells look like cells of origin	Tumour usually not encapsulated Metastasis possible Necrosis within tumour Cells and nuclei are non-uniform Tissue of origin may be not recognisable from the appearance of the tumour cells
Uniform mitotic figures Arrangement of tumour cells may look similar to the normal tissue of origin	Abnormal or irregular mitotic figures Tumour usually does not retain recognisable tissue architecture

4. a. Metastasis is:

   The spread of malignant tumour from its site of origin (primary tumour) to form a secondary tumour, also called a *metastasis*.

   b. Three means by which tumours metastasise.
      Choose from:
      i. haematogenous spread
      ii. lymphatic spread
      iii. serosal spread
      iv. intra-organ spread

5. Short notes to discuss two of the ways a tumour exerts harmful effects.

   Choose two of the following:

   Physical presence of the tumour – e.g. abnormal presence of a growing mass. Malignant or benign tumours may be harmful merely because of their position. So, a tumour in the lungs may cause coughing or breathlessness, a mass in the stomach may stimulate vomiting whilst one in the urinary bladder may lead to inability to urinate. Brain tumours press on the brain as they grow within the rigid skull.

   Bleeding and infection – ulcerated, infected or highly vascular tumours may provide evidence of their presence in an organ because of blood, bacteria or inflammatory cells in sputum, vomit or urine.

   Pain – tumours may cause pain due to pressure on, or invasion into, other organs, e.g. invasion of bone by tumour is very painful.

   Weight loss – loss of body condition or wasting in animals with tumours may be secondary to nausea, vomiting or inappetence. Marked wasting (cachexia) is also a primary effect of tumours and is due to the tumour-secreting chemical messengers which increase muscle breakdown (catabolism).

   Effects of chemical messengers (other than catabolism) – non-specific signs such as fever (*pyrexia of unknown origin*, or PUO) or anaemia or leukopenia (decreased white blood cell count) due to inhibition of bone marrow.

   Change in haematology – changes in the blood profile, such as increased neutrophils, may occur in tumours which become infected. In some cases the animal's response to infection will be inhibited by effects of the tumour on the bone marrow. Blood clotting may also be adversely affected due to bone marrow inhibition, but also to any effects the tumour may have on liver function and decrease in clotting factors.

Inappropriate hormone secretion – many tumour cells retain the functions of their normal cell of origin, but fail to respond to normal control mechanisms. Thus, in the case of tumours derived from a hormone-secreting cell of an endocrine organ, for instance, the cells may secrete inappropriately high levels of hormone. Thus, tumours of the pituitary gland of elderly dogs can lead to a form of *hyperadrenocorticism* or Cushing's disease by secondary over-stimulation of the adrenal cortex.

Alternatively, the tumour mass may be composed of neoplastic cells that are not 'functionally active' (i.e. do not produce hormone). The growing mass of inactive tumour cells presses on adjacent normal cells in the endocrine organ causing them to atrophy or die (necrosis). Eventually, the function of the tissue is reduced because the inactive tumour cells take up more space than normal active endocrine cells (*space-occupying* effect). This is at least partially responsible for the complex effects of Cushing's disease in older horses, thought to be partially due to pressure of a growing tumour on the overlying area of brain (the hypothalamus) which regulates body temperature, appetite and hair shedding.

6. Discussion of cytology in the diagnosis of neoplasms in veterinary general practice.

Cytology is a useful early step in diagnosis, being relatively cheap, easy and non-invasive. Good quality smears are useful for assessing some cell features and may allow rapid diagnosis or at least might indicate that further procedures (such as biopsy) are warranted.

Cytology may also be used in practice to investigate whether the tumour has spread to another site, e.g. a local lymph node.

Cytological techniques used in general practice include thin smears on glass microscope slides of samples – fine-needle aspirates (FNAs), which may be gently sucked with a syringe (aspirated) from the middle of the tumour. FNAs may also be made from body or tissue fluids such as bronchiolar lavage (BAL – washed from the trachea), urine or peritoneal tap fluids. Finally, a tumour or part of a tumour may be dabbed on to the glass slide to produce impression smears of tissues.

All these preparations may be air-dried, stained and examined under the microscope in the practice laboratory, though the dried slides may also be sent to a clinical pathologist.

Further Reading

There are many books which might be helpful to take you further into veterinary pathology than this one. Below are a few suggestions, but do not limit yourself to these if you find you have caught the pathology bug!

An Introduction to General Pathology, by Tim D. Spector and John S. Axford, Churchill Livingstone; 4th edition (1999).

Cell, Tissue and Disease: The Basis of Pathology, by Neville Woolf, W.B. Saunders; 3rd edition (2000).

Clinical Immunology of the Dog and Cat, by Michael J. Day, Manson Publishing Ltd; 2nd edition (2008).

Introduction to Veterinary Pathology, by Norman F. Cheville, Wiley-Blackwell; 2nd edition (1999).

Thomson's Special Veterinary Pathology, by M. Donald McGavin, William W. Carlton, James F. Zachary, Mosby; 3rd revised edition (2000).

Veterinary Immunology: An Introduction, by Ian R. Tizard, Saunders; 8th edition (2008).

Index

abscess, abscessation, 13, 32, 55, 56, 159, 190
accumulation, of substances in cells, 26, 28, 38
acid–base levels of blood, 149
acidosis, 149
acquired coagulopathy, 138
acquired diseases, 15, 190
acquired immune system/response, adaptive
    immune system/response, specific immune
    system/response, 67, 69–84, 190, 210
acute inflammation, 42, 43–55, 61, 63, 79, 80,
    103, 190
    cardinal or clinical, signs, 43, 44, 47, 49
adaptations of cells, 154
adenocarcinoma, 159, 160, 190
adhesion, 55, 56
adrenal cortex, 177
adrenocorticotropic hormone, ACTH, 15, 109,
    177
aetiologic agent(s), or factors, 12–18, 190
aetiology, 12, 13
age or aging, 15, 19, 36–8, 87, 109, 145–56
alanine aminotransferase, AAT, 31
albumin, 50
allantoin, 36, 37
allergen, 55, 56, 90
allergy, allergic reactions, 62, 90, 91, 93, 190
amyloid, 36, 37, 38
anaemia, anaemic, 6, 8, 28, 51, 53, 63, 69, 88,
    93, 155, 156, 176, 180, 190
anaesthetics, 115
anal sac (adeno)carcinoma, 178, 179
anaphylactic shock, anaphylaxis, 91, 190, 191
anasarca, 126, 191
anatomic pathology, 4, 191
angiogenesis, 137, 167–9
annular growth, 172
anorexia, 53
antibiotics, 6
antibody, antibodies, see also
    immunoglobulins, 7, 59, 63, 69, 72–8, 81,
    83–6, 88–92, 114, 183, 191
antibody complexes, 91, 92, 191
antibody/immunoglobin classes, 75, 78
anticoagulant (rodent poison), 8
antifreeze, 36, 37
antigen, antigenicity, 7, 69, 72–83, 85, 86, 90,
    92, 183, 191

antigen binding site, of
    antibody/immunoglobin, see also variable
    region of antibody (immunoglobulin), 72,
    74
antigen presenting cells, 78, 79, 81, 83, 85, 86
antimicrobial factors, of neutrophils, 51
aorta, 116–18, 144
apoptosis, 191
appetite loss, inappetence, 53, 56, 176, 180
arterial bleeds, 116
arteriolar circulation/supply, 116, 117, 148
arteriole, 45, 47, 116, 117, 119, 129, 139
artery, arteries, 116, 117, 119
ascites, 126, 191
asthma, 91
atrium, atria, of heart, 116, 120
atrophy, 38, 62, 93, 154–6, 180, 191
autoimmune disease, autoimmunity, 69, 93, 94,
    191
autoimmune haemolytic anaemia, AIHA, 93
autolysis, autolyse, 30, 182, 191
automated blood analyser, 4
autonomic nervous system, 149

B cells/lymphocytes, 70, 72–6, 81, 83, 85, 86,
    92
bacteraemia, 191
bacterial capsule, 60
bacterium/bacteria, 6, 12–15, 30, 32–5, 44, 50,
    51, 60, 66–9, 79, 81, 104, 109, 166, 176,
    192
bandage, or dressing, 4, 30, 125, 154
basophil, 192
bee sting, 127
'bends', the, 145
benign tumour, 157, 167, 169–71, 183, 192
Bernese mountain dog, 166
bile pigments, 28, 38
bile, 28, 36, 37
biliary tract, 186
bilirubin, 38
biochemistry of blood, 87
biopsy, 4, 5, 181, 182, 192
birds, 36, 37
bitch, bitches, 87, 156
Black Death, the, 14
bladder, urinary, 36, 37, 38, 155

bleeding, *see also* blood in specific situations, e.g. urine, blood in, 32, 180
blister, blistering, *see also* vesicle, 93
blood, 87, 88, 114, 115, 146, 147, 179, 181
    coagulation, clotting, *see also* coagulation cascade, haemostasis, 75, 132–7, 177, 180, 192
    groups, 192
    transfusions, 69
body temperature, 177
bone, 9, 137, 139, 145, 159, 174, 176, 178–80
bone marrow, 51, 53, 57, 59, 62, 63, 72, 77, 81, 88, 100, 139, 145, 155, 156, 159, 176, 177, 180
brain, 31, 33, 50, 53, 109, 126, 148, 149, 166, 176
breathlessness, 93
breed-specific tumours, 166
broncho-alveolar lavage, BAL, 181
bubonic plague, 14
burn(s), 44, 138

cachexia, 176, 180
calcification, 35, 37, 192
    dystrophic, 35, 37, 38, 195
    metastatic, 35, 37, 38, 203
calcium oxalate, 36, 38
calcium, 35, 37, 132, 133, 178, 179
calculi, or liths, 35–8, 155, 157
calor, 44
cancer, 44, 157
canine distemper virus, CDV, 87
canine genome project, the, 166
canine infectious respiratory disease, CIRD, 19, 20
capillary (bed), capillaries, 45–9, 115–21, 146–8, 167, 168
capsule, fibrous, of tumour, 169, 170
carbon, 28, 38
carbon dioxide, 116
carcinogen, 160, 166, 192
carcinogenesis, 160, 192
carcinoma, 145, 160, 192
cardiac muscle, 100
cardinal or clinical, signs of acute inflammation, 43, 44, 47, 49
cardinal signs of acute inflammation, 43, 44, 159
cardiogenic shock, 148, 192
cartilage, 159
caseation necrosis, 31, 34, 38, 193
cat(s), 13, 28, 61, 87, 88, 93, 130, 139, 142, 144, 155, 156
catabolic effects of tumours, 176
cattle, 139, 166
cell(s), 2, 3, 18
    cycle, 161–5
    differentiation, 161, 165, 193
    proliferation, 161
cell-mediated immunity/immune response, 70, 81, 82, 193
cellular degeneration, 26, 38
cellular exudate, 50, 54
cellular phase of acute inflammation, 44, 50, 56, 77
cellulitis, 32, 35
Celsus, 43
cervical cancer, 166, 181
checkpoints, of cell cycle, 163–5

chemical factors, in pathogenesis, 15, 44, 137, 166
chemical messengers/mediators, 46, 50, 51, 53, 57, 59, 61, 67, 68, 81, 82, 92, 114, 162, 167, 176, 180
chemotherapy, 110
cholera outbreak, London, 14
cholestasis, 193
chronic inflammation, 42, 43, 55, 58–61, 63, 155, 157, 166, 193
cilia, 67, 68
circulation, blood, 57, 109, 116
classification of diseases, 15
clinical pathology, chemical pathology, clinical pathologist, 4, 181, 193
clone of cells, 75, 157, 158
clotting factors, 132, 133, 139, 177, 180
cloudy swelling, 193
coagulation cascade, *see also* blood clotting, haemostasis, blood coagulation, 132–5, 193
coagulative necrosis, 30, 33, 38, 193
coagulopathy, coagulopathies, 138, 139, 194
    acquired, 138
    congenital, 138
colitis, 43
collagen, 103, 194
collagenous, 194
colliquative necrosis, 31, 33
colostrum, 88, 89
complement cascade, complement proteins, 75, 77, 79, 80, 85–7, 92
compression, as cause of ischaemia, 30, 128
congenital disease/condition, 16, 17, 194
conjunctivitis, 93
constipation, 172
consumption coagulopathy, 137, 138, 194
cornified layer, of skin, 67
corticosteroids, 19, 88
coughing, with tumours, 176
creatine kinase, CK, 31
crepitus, crepitant feel to tissues, 32, 35, 194
cross-linking of fibrin, 133, 135
cruelty (forensic pathology), 8
crystallisation, crystal formation, 36–8
culture and sensitivity, 6
Cushing's disease, 15, 177
cutaneous histiocytoma, 166, 178
cytokine, 81, 82, 84, 92, 194
cytology, 6, 181, 194
cytotoxic, 79, 194
    hypersensitivity, 92, 194
    T cells, 79, 81–3, 85

Dalmation dogs, 36, 37
deep vein thrombosis, DVT, 141
degeneration, cellular, 26, 38, 195
degranulation, 46, 48, 50, 52, 55, 56, 61, 90, 91, 195
dehydration, 147
delayed type hypersensitivity, 92, 195
demodex, 7, 87
demolition phase of organisation healing, 101, 102
dendritic cells, 70, 78, 79, 83, 85, 86, 195
denervation, 110
dental plaque, dental disease, 35, 37, 155, 156
de-oxygenated blood, 117

de-oxyribonucleic acid, DNA, 14, 162–5
depression, 149
dermal fibroma, 160
dermatitis, 9, 28, 43, 93,
developmental abnormalities, 16
diabetes mellitus, 15, 28, 109
diagnosis, 181,
diarrhoea, 4, 61, 126
dicoumarol, 138
diet, 87
differentiation of cells, 100, 161
dipstick for testing urine, 4
Dirofilaria, heartworm, 145
disease
    acquired, 15
    classification of, 15
    congenital, 16, 17
    hereditary, 17
    idiopathic, 16, 199
    modifiers of development, 16
    multifactorial, 16, 19, 20
    simple, 16, 18
    treatment of, 19
    vulnerability to, 16, 19
disseminated, 195
    intravascular coagulation, DIC, 137, 138, 146,
        195
division phase of cell cycle, 156
dog(s), 5, 36, 37, 87, 93, 104, 108, 139, 145,
        165, 166, 178, 186
dolor, 44
dome (tumour growth), 169, 170
draft animals, 31, 34
drugs, 88, 93
dry gangrene, 32, 35, 195
dystrophic calcification, 35, 37, 38, 192

ecchymoses, 140, 195
effusion, 195
eggs, ova, 162, 165,
electrolytes (salts), 50, 114, 122
electron microscope, 183
embolism, 128, 142, 144, 145
embolus, 142–5, 195
    fat, 145
    fibrocartilage, 145
    gas, 145
    infective/inflammatory, 145
    parasitic, 145
    tumour, 145
endogenous, 28, 195
endothelium, endothelial cells, 46, 48, 52, 90,
        100, 115, 119, 127, 132–5, 138, 139, 146,
        195
endotoxin, 141
enteritis, 43, 61
environmental factors and disease, 14, 19, 20
enzyme(s), 31, 33, 36, 37, 46, 54, 62, 75, 79, 80,
        132, 133
eosinophil(s), 55, 56, 61, 62, 91, 101, 195
    horse, 62
eosinophilic granuloma complex, EGC, 61,
        92
epicardium, *see also* pericardium, 174
epidermis, 93, 100, 102–7
epithelium, epithelial cells, 62, 67, 68, 93, 100,
        103–7, 159, 160
erosion, 32, 93, 169, 171, 172, 180, 182,
        196

erythrocytes, *see also* red blood cells, 6
ethylene glycol, 36, 37
evidence, handling of (forensic pathology), 8
excision margins, 6, 182, 196
excisional biopsy, 5, 181, 196
exogenous, 28, 196
external factors and disease, 15
extracellular changes/accumulations, 32, 35, 36,
        38
extrinsic pathway of blood clotting, 132, 133
exudate, 46, 49, 50, 90, 104, 109, 159, 175,
        176, 196
    cellular, 50
    fibrinous, 54
    haemorrhagic, 54
    mucopurulent, 54
    necrohaemorrhagic, 54
    purulent, 54
    serous, 54
    suppurative, 54, 55, 210
exudative phase of acute inflammation, 44, 46,
        56
eye, 93

face, 61
factor VIII, 139
faeces, blood in, 172
farm animals, 8
fat necrosis, 31, 34, 38
fat(s), 28, 31, 67, 68
fatty change, 28, 38, 196
feline immunodeficiency virus, FIV, 87, 88
feline infectious peritonitis, FIP, 59, 61, 87, 91,
        92, 138
feline leukaemia virus, FeELV, 87, 88, 166,
        181
fever, 50, 53, 54, 56, 63, 180
fibrin, 54–6, 103, 104, 132–7, 145, 196
fibrinogen, 50, 132–7, 196
fibrinolysis, 134–7
fibrinous exudate, 54
fibroblasts, 60, 102
fibrocartilage, 145
fibrosis, fibrous tissue, *see also* scar, scarring,
        scar tissue, 55, 59, 60, 62, 63, 98, 99,
        101–4, 109, 130, 131, 159, 169, 170,
        196
fine-needle aspirate, FNA, 5, 6, 181
first intention healing, 104, 106
fleas, 4, 7
flock health, 8
food allergies, 91
food quality and safety (human health), 8
foreign material, and chronic inflammation, 57,
        58, 60, 61, 145
'foreign' molecules, and immune responses, 67,
        68
forensic pathology, veterinary, 8
formalin, 5
formalin-fixed tissue, 5, 181, 182
formol saline, 5
functio laesa, 44
functional changes, 24, 25, 26, 61
functionally (endocrinologically) active tumours,
        177
fungus/fungi, 6, 12, 14, 15, 44, 66

Galen, 43
gallstones, 38

gangrene, 31, 35, 38, 146, 196
  dry, 32, 35, 38, 195
  gas, 32, 35, 38, 196
  moist, 32, 35, 38, 203
  wet, 32, 35, 38, 213
gap phases of cell cycle, 162
gas gangrene, 32, 35, 38, 195
general pathology, 9, 197
genes, 14, 16, 17, 19, 197
genetic abnormalities/mutations, of tumours,
  15, 19, 157, 158, 161, 165
genetic disease/condition, 14, 15, 197
globulins, 50, 63, 87, 197
glucocorticoids, *see also* corticosteroids, 88
glycoprotein, 105, 119, 139
goats, 93
golden retriever, 4, 16
gout, articular, renal and visceral, 36–8
government agency laboratories, 8
granulation tissue, granulation phase of
  organisation, 101–4, 197
granuloma(s), 59–61, 63, 166, 197
granulomatous inflammation, 58–63, 92, 145,
  197
growth factors, 109, 114, 162
growth hormone, 166
growth-inhibiting factors, of cell cycle,
  163–5
growth-promoting factors, of cell cycle,
  163–5
gum(s), 35, 37
gut(s), (intestine), 38, 43, 55, 59, 155, 156

haemangioma/haemangiosarcoma, 167
haematocrit, 197
haematogenous spread of tumour, 174, 175
haematology, 6, 51, 53, 63, 87, 177, 180, 197
haematoma, 140, 197
haematopoietic tissue, 100, 159
haematoxylin and eosin, H and E (histology
  stains), 5
haemoconcentration, 197
haemolysis, 198
haemopericardium, haemothorax,
  haemoperitoneum, 140, 198
haemophillia A, 139
haemorrhage, 32, 54, 134, 137–40, 147, 198
haemorrhagic exudate, 54
haemosiderin, 28, 38
haemostasis, 134, 135, 141
  primary, 134, 135
  secondary, 134, 135
hair coat, 177
harmful effects of acute inflammation, 54
harmful effects of chronic inflammation, 61
harness(es), 31, 34
hay fever, 46, 49, 90
healing
  by first intention or primary union, 104, 106
  by secondary intention or secondary union,
    104, 107
heart, 30, 45, 108, 115–17, 125, 130, 141, 144,
  148, 155, 156
heart disease, heart failure, 142, 148
heartworm, *Dirofilaria* sp., 145
heavy chains, of antibodies/immunoglobins,
  72–5, 78
heavy metals, 15
Helicobacter sp., 166

hepatitis, 43
herd health, 8
hereditary disease or condition, 17, 198
histamine, 46, 48, 198
histiocytoma, 166, 178
histiosarcoma, 166
histology, 5, 181
histopathology, 90, 198
hormones, 87, 114, 149, 155, 156, 165, 166,
  177, 180
horse(s), 31, 34, 87, 93, 110, 139, 177, 185
  eosinophil, 62
human health, human diseases, 8, 36, 37, 46,
  49, 88, 90, 106, 141, 166, 181, 186
human immunodeficiency virus, HIV, AIDS, 88
human papilloma virus, HPV, 106, 181
humor, 14, 81
humoral immunity/immune response, 70, 81,
  82, 198
hydropericardium, hydrothorax, 126, 198
hydropic change, 28, 38
hydrostatic pressure, 122, 123, 125, 198
hygiene, 14, 15, 19, 69
hyperadrenocorticism, HAC, 15, 10, 177
hyperaemia, 46, 47, 198
hypercalcaemia, 178, 179
hypercoagulability, of blood, 141, 198
hyperplasia, 38, 58, 59, 154–7, 198
hypersensitivity, hypersensitivities, 44, 55, 56,
  60–62, 78, 89–93, 148, 198
hypertrophic cardiomyopathy, 142, 144, 155,
  156
hypertrophy, 38, 59, 108, 154–6, 199
hypoglycaemia, 149
hypothalamus, 177
hypovolaemia, 146, 147, 199
hypovolaemic shock, 146, 147, 199
hypoxia, 132, 149

iatrogenic, 199
icterus, 199
idiopathic, disease, 16, 28, 61, 199
iliac arteries, 142, 144
immediate hypersensitivity, 90, 199
immune complexes, 92
immune response (system), 7, 42, 44, 55–7,
  59–61, 63, 66–96, 166, 172, 173, 178, 183,
  199
immunity, 19, 20, 199
immunocompromise, 178, 199
immunodeficiency, immunodeficiencies, 66, 84,
  109, 199
immunogen, immunogenic, 69
immunoglobulin(s), 72–6, 78, 83, 85, 87, 88,
  199
immunoglobin/antibody classes, 75, 78
  immunoglobin A, 75, 78
  immunoglobin D, 78
  immunoglobin E, 78
  immunoglobin G, 75, 78
  immunoglobin M, 78
immunology, 7, 199
immunostaining, immunohistochemistry, 7, 183,
  200
immunostains, 7
immunosuppression, 69, 87, 200
impression smear, of tumour, 181
incisional biopsy, 5, 181, 200
incubation period, 200

infarction, 55, 56, 127–32, 141, 142, 156, 167, 200
    focal, 129, 130
    global, 129, 130
infected wound, 4
infectious agents or organisms, 6, 7, 12, 14, 16, 19, 20, 60, 67, 68, 72, 74, 137, 145
infectious canine hepatitis virus, ICH, 138
inflammation, 9, 13, 32, 33, 42, 67, 68, 78, 85, 86, 90, 92, 134, 137, 145, 171, 200
inflammatory border, of infarct, 130, 131
inflammatory oedema, 122, 124
inflammatory phase of healing, 101, 102
initiation (in tumour formation), 160, 161, 166, 200
innate immune system, 67, 68, 82, 84, 85, 200
insect, 61
intercellular junction, 46, 49, 50, 115, 119
internal factors and disease, 15
interstitial fluid, 115, 118, 120, 121, 167, 200
interstitium, 115, 118, 120, 122, 123, 200
intestine, intestinal tract (gut), 36, 43, 55, 59, 67, 68, 78, 100, 131, 132, 138, 149, 159, 172
intracytoplasmic granules, 46, 48, 51, 57, 61, 62, 84, 90, 134, 135
intra-organ spread of tumour, 175, 176
intra-venous injections, 145
intrinsic pathway, of blood clotting, 132, 133
intussusception, 201
invasion (of tumour growth), 169, 171, 182, 183, 185, 201
irreversible (non-reversible) cell change/damage/injury, 24, 26, 38, 98, 99, 154, 157, 201
ischaemia, ischaemic necrosis, 44, 55, 56, 108, 127–32, 137, 141, 142, 148, 156, 167, 201
isotypes of immunoglobulins, 72, 78,
itchy (skin), 4
-itis, 42, 43

jaundice, 28, 69, 201

kennel cough, 19
keratinisation, 201
kidney, 30, 35–8, 43, 130, 149
    (renal) failure, 35–7, 100, 108
kittens, 88

labile cells, 99–101, 103, 104, 155, 156, 162, 201
lactation, 20, 155, 156
large granular lymphocytes, 84, 201
larvae, parasites, 145
larynx, 127
latent period, 201
lead walking of dogs, 104
leakiness of capillaries, 46, 48–50, 56, 115, 118, 124
'left shift', of neutrophils, 51, 53
lesion(s), 24, 25, 201
lethargy, 149
leucocytes, 6, 44, 50, 52, 145, 201
leucopenia, 176, 180
leukaemia, 88, 201
light chains, of antibodies/immunoglobins, 72–5
lip, 61
liquefactive necrosis, 31, 33, 34, 201
liths, or calculi, 35–8, 155, 157

liver, 3, 24, 25, 28, 31, 36, 37, 43, 100, 108, 131–3, 138, 155–7, 174, 175, 177, 180
long-term (chronic) disease(s), 61
lungs, 29, 36, 45, 100, 108, 115, 130–132, 138, 141, 145, 149, 174–6
lymph, 120, 201
lymph nodes, 72, 75, 77, 81, 85, 120, 159, 174, 175, 182
lymphadenopathy, 202
lymphatic spread of tumour, 174, 175
lymphocytes, 55–60, 63, 67–79, 81–8, 92, 101, 178, 202
lymphoid circulation, lymphatic circulation, 49, 115, 116, 118, 120, 122, 125, 172–6
lymphoid organs/tissue, 79, 81, 83, 85, 100, 125
lymphoma, lymphoid tumours, 160, 166, 178, 179
lymphopenia, 88
lysis and resolution of thrombus, 143
lysosomes, 202

macrophages, 55, 57, 59, 60, 63, 67–71, 78, 81, 83, 85–8, 92, 101, 102, 141, 178, 179, 202
malacia, 31, 33
malaise, 53
malicious harm (forensic pathology), 8
malignant calcification, 35, 37, 38
malignant melanoma, 160
malignant tumour, malignancy, 157, 160, 161, 167, 169, 171–6, 178, 183–5, 202
mammary adenocarcinoma/tumour, 145, 160, 166, 169, 174
mammary gland, 78, 155, 156, 160
margination, 50, 52
margins, of tumours, 169, 171, 182
mast cells, 45, 46, 48, 49, 55, 56, 77, 80, 90, 91, 148, 202
masticatory myopathy, 93
maturation phase of healing/organisation, 101, 102
mediators, chemical, 46, 50, 51, 53, 57, 59, 61, 67, 68, 114
megakaryocytes, 134, 139
melaena, 140, 202
melanin, 28, 36
'memory' in immune response, 67, 75, 77, 81, 85
memory T cells (memory cells), 81, 82, 202
meningitis, 31, 33
mesenchymal cells, 159, 160
metabolism, metabolic activity/characteristics of tissues, 28, 36, 109, 149
metaplasia, 38, 62, 154–7, 202
metastasis, 167, 169, 171–6, 180, 182–4, 202
metastatic calcification, 35, 37, 203
'met' (metastasis) check, of tumours, 172
microbiology, 6, 87, 203
micrometastasis, 185
microscope(s), 7, 14, 29, 62, 176, 178, 181, 182
microtome, 5
mineral, 35–8
mineralisation, 35, 37
mink, 36, 37
mitosis, 100, 103, 104, 156, 162, 183, 203
mitotic figures, 183, 184
mitotic index, 183
modifiers (in disease development), 16
modifiers (in tumour formation), 166, 167
moist gangrene, 32, 35

monocytes, 57, 70, 203
mononuclear cells, 59
mosquito, 61
motile, motility of cells, 50, 51, 62
muco-cutaneous junctions, 93
mucopurulent exudate, 54
mucous membranes, 66, 69, 149
mucus, 6, 36, 37, 67, 68, 85
multifactorial disease, 16, 19, 20, 203
multinucleated giant cells, 57–60
muscle(s), 31, 62, 93, 100, 131, 132, 149, 154,
    156, 165, 176, 180
muscular dystrophy, 16
mutation (genetic), 15, 19, 157, 158, 161, 164,
    203
myalgia, 53
mycologist(s), 6

naïve animal, 19
native immune system, natural immune system,
    67, 68, 82, 84–6, 203
natural killer cells, 67, 68, 82, 84–6, 203
nausea, 53, 176, 180
necrohaemorrhagic exudate, 54
necropsy, 4, 8, 203
necrosis, 26, 30–36, 44, 98, 99, 103, 127, 138,
    148, 167, 170, 171, 177, 180, 183, 204
neoplasia, 9, 88, 157–86, 204
neoplasm(s), 157–86, 204
neoplastic cells, 115
nephritis, 61
nerves, 100, 108, 148, 155, 156
nervous tissue/system, 108, 109
neurogenic shock, 148, 204
neurones, 100
neutropenia, 204
neutrophil(s), 13, 50–57, 60, 62, 63, 67, 68, 87,
    88, 92, 101, 102, 104, 141, 177, 180, 204
neutrophilia, 204
nodular, 204
    liver regeneration, 108, 157
non-granulomatous inflammation, 58, 59, 63
non-inflammatory oedema, 124, 125
non-reversible cell damage, see also
    irreversible cell damage, 98, 99
'non-self' and immune response, 69
nose, 61
noxious, 204
nutrition (role in pathogenesis), 14, 155, 156
nutrition (role in wound healing), 109

oedema, 90, 120, 122–7, 141, 204
    dependent, 126
    generalised, 126
    inflammatory, 122, 124
    localised, 126
    non-inflammatory, 124
    pulmonary, 126
oesophagus, 166
-oma, 159, 204
oncogenesis, 205
oncology, 186
-opathy, 205
ophthalmoscope, 140
organisation, 55, 56, 98, 99, 101–4, 106–9, 130,
    131, 205
osmotic activity, 122, 123
osmotic pressure, 120, 123, 125, 126
osteoclasts, 178, 179

osteosarcoma, 9, 160, 166
oxen, 31, 34
oxygen, 28, 116, 127, 132, 167, 168
oxygen free radicals, 46, 49, 205
oxygenated blood, 116, 117

pain, 13, 43, 44, 51, 53, 56, 62, 149, 176, 180
pallor, 93, 130, 131
pancreas, 35, 186
pancreatitis, 31, 34, 37
pancytopenia, 205
papillary, of tumour growth, 169, 170
papillomavirus, 106, 181
paraffin wax block (in histology), 5
paraneoplastic effect/syndrome, 177–80, 205
parasite(s), 6, 7, 15, 44, 60–62, 78, 166, 205
parasitology, 6
parathyroid hormone, 35, 37, 178, 179
parathyroid hormone related peptide, PHrP
    (parathyroid-like hormone), 35, 37, 178,
    179
passive immunity, 88, 89, 205
patch test, for allergy, 93
pathogen(s), 12, 84, 114, 206
pathogenesis, 12, 13, 206
pathogenic factor, 206
pathognomonic, 206
pathologists, vii, 3–10, 174, 181, 182
pathology, vii, viii, 2, 206
pedunculated, of tumour growth, 169, 170
pemphigus complex of skin diseases, 93
perfusion, 206
pericarditis, suppurative, 55, 56
pericardium, 55, 56
peritoneal tap, 181
peritoneum, 31, 54–6, 174
peritonitis, 55
peritonitis, suppurative, 55, 56
permanent cells, 99, 100, 103, 109, 163, 206
permeability, of capillaries, see also vascular
    permeability, 146, 147
petechiae, 140, 206
pH, of blood, 149
phagocytosis, phagocytic cells, phagocytic
    cells, 51, 57, 58, 62, 67, 68, 70, 77, 79, 80,
    92, 141, 206
pharmaceutical laboratories, 8
pharmacological substances, 115
phase of DNA production of cell cycle, 162
physical barriers, in body, 67, 68
physical factors (in pathogenesis), 15
physiologic stresses, 20, 87
pigments, 28, 38
pigs, 89, 127
pinch biopsy, 206
pituitary, 177
plaque (of tumour growth), 169, 170
plaques, dental, 35, 37, 38
plasma, 206
    cells, 55, 59, 60, 63, 69–71, 74–7, 83, 85, 86,
        88, 101, 206
    proteins, 50, 67, 68, 122, 123, 126, 207
plaster cast, 156
platelets, 50, 114, 132–5, 139, 141, 207
pleura, 54, 55, 56, 174,
pleural adhesions, 55
pleurisy, 207
pneumonia, 15, 55, 207
poison(s), 8, 15, 17

police involvement (forensic pathology), 8
pollen grains, 90
pollution, 28
portosystemic shunt, 156
pregnancy, 16, 17, 20, 87, 93, 155, 156
pressure (in pathogenesis), 15
primary immunodeficiency, 84, 207
primary tumour, 169, 173–6
primary union, healing by, 104, 106
'priming' of immune cells, 84
production animals, 8
prognosis, 87, 160, 165, 174, 178, 181, 186, 207
progression, of tumour development, 161, 164, 165
promotion of tumour development, promoters, 161, 166
prostate specific antigen, PSA, 186
prostate tumours, 174, 186
proteases, 50, 51
protective role, of inflammation, 42, 43, 54, 79, 85
protein(s), 29, 31, 36, 38, 49, 60, 63, 67, 68, 75, 79–81, 90, 93, 103, 114
proud flesh, 110
pruritus, 91, 207
pulmonary artery, 116, 117
    embolism, 141
    pulmonary vein, 116, 117
punch biopsy, 207
puppy, puppies, 87, 88, 156
purulent exudate, 54
purulent, 207
pus, 6, 13, 32, 54, 207
putrefactive, 32, 35,
pyo-, 208
pyogranulomatous, inflammation, 59, 91, 92
pyrexia of unknown origin, PUO, 176, 180

quiescent, 208

rabbits, hypothetical!, 17
radiation, 15, 44, 110, 166
radiographs, 172, 181, 182
reactive, 208
recanalisation, of thrombus, 142, 208
recruitment of leukocytes, 50, 52
red blood cells, 6, 28, 50, 52, 53, 54, 63, 93
regeneration, of tissues/cells, 32, 98–101, 103, 108, 109, 130, 131, 208, 211
regenerative capacity, of cells/tissues, 32, 98, 100, 103
regression of tumours, 178
renal (kidney) failure, 35, 36, 37
repair, 208
reproductive tract, 66
respiratory rate, in shock, 149
respiratory tract, 67, 68, 78, 159
resting phase of cell cycle, 162
retinal haemorrhages, 140
retroviruses, 166, 208
reversible cell change/damage/injury, 24, 38, 154, 208
road traffic accident, RTA, 145, 156
rodenticides, rodent poisons, 8, 138
roundworm, in horses, 44
rubor, 44

'saddle' thrombus, cats, 142, 144

saliva, 35
Salmonella, 138
salt poisoning and brain oedema, 126
salts, see also sodium chloride, 50, 114, 122, 123
sarcoma, 159, 160, 166, 208
scab, 103–7
scar/scar tissue, see also fibrosis, fibrous tissue, fibrovascular tissue, 32, 55, 56, 62, 99, 101, 102, 104–8, 130, 131, 142, 208
sclerosis, 208
sebaceous adenoma, 160
sebum, 67
second intention healing, secondary union, 104, 107
secondary immunodeficiency, 87, 209
secondary infection, 13, 169
secondary tumour, 169, 173–6
segmented or multilobed nuclei, 51, 62
'self' and immune responses, 13, 69, 72, 93
self-trauma/self-harm, 42, 43, 54, 56, 109, 209
sensitivity, bacterial (to antibiotics), 6
septic, 209
    shock, 55, 56, 146, 148, 209
septicaemia, 138, 209
sequela(e), 32, 209
sequestration, 32
serology, 7, 209
serosal spread/seeding of tumour, 174–6
serous exudate, 54
serum, 7, 54, 56, 78, 103, 209
severe combined immunodeficiency, SCID, 87
'shelling out', of tumours, 169, 170, 182
'shift to the left' of neutrophils, 51, 53
shivering, in shock, 149
shock, 91, 145–50, 209
    cardiogenic, 148
    clinical signs of, 149
    neurogenic, 148
    psychological, 145
    septic or toxic, 55, 56, 146, 148, 209, 211
shunt, 156
signalment, 182
simple disease, 16, 18, 210
skin, 4, 9, 13, 28, 36, 43, 55, 56, 59, 61, 66–8, 78, 87, 91, 93, 103–7, 137, 149, 159, 166
'skip' metastases, 174, 175
sludging of capillaries, 149
smallpox, 14
snake(s), 35, 37, 138
sodium chloride, 123
solutes, osmotically active, 123
somatic cells, 162
space-occupying effect of tumour, 177, 180
special pathology, 9, 210
sperm, 162, 165
spinal cord, 109
spinal injuries, 109
spleen, 72, 75, 79, 81, 93, 137, 139, 174, 175
splinters, 60, 61
sputum, blood in, 172, 176, 180
stable cells, 99–101, 103, 155, 156, 162, 210
stem cell, 70, 82, 100, 101, 103, 210
stimuli, harmful, 24, 28, 43, 44
stomach cancer, 166, 176
stomach contents (for toxicology), 8
strongyle infection, in horses, 130
structural changes, 24–6, 61
sub-cellular, of study of pathology, 2, 3

suckling, 88, 89
sunlight, 166
suppuration, 62, 210
suppurative, exudate, 54, 55, 56, 210
sutures, stitches, 60, 61, 104
sympathetic nervous system, 149
syndrome, 210
systemic, 210
   effects of acute inflammation, 50, 53, 54
   pathology, 9, 210

T cells/lymphocytes, 70, 72, 77–9, 81–6
T helper cells, 74, 79, 81–3, 85, 86, 91, 92
tachycardia, 93
tattoo inks, 29, 38
terminal differentiation phase of cell cycle, 163
tertiary or third stage tumours, 172
testes, 186
   Test yourself questions, on Chapter 1, 10
   Test yourself questions, on Chapter 2, 21
   Test yourself questions, on Chapter 3, 39
   Test yourself questions, on Chapter 4, 64
   Test yourself questions, on Chapter 5, 95
   Test yourself questions, on Chapter 6, 111
   Test yourself questions, on Chapter 7, 151
   Test yourself questions, on Chapter 8, 188
thromboembolism, 141, 210
thromboembolus, thromboemboli, 142, 143, 210
thrombosis, 55, 56, 128, 211
thrombus, 131, 134, 140–142, 211
thymus, 59, 72, 77, 81
tissue processing, 5
tissue repair, 211
tissue transplant, 69
tobacco smoke, 166
torsion, 211
toxaemia, 211
toxic shock, 146, 211
toxicologist(s), 8
toxicology, 7, 211
toxin, 8, 15, 24, 25, 46, 49, 108, 114, 138, 146, 148, 155, 156, 211
trachea, 159, 175, 176, 181
transformation of cells, 157–9, 161, 162, 165, 166, 169, 211
transudate, 211
trauma, 15, 44, 87
treatment, 19
tuberculosis, 31, 34, 60, 61
tumor, 43, 44, 159
tumour(s), 5, 7, 35, 62, 137, 157–86, 211
   angiogenesis factor, TAF, 167, 168
   cells, 69, 81, 84
   growth patterns, 169–72
   initiation, 200
   markers, 183, 186, 212
   progression, 161, 164, 165
   promotion, 161, 166
type I hypersensitivity reaction, 90, 91, 212
type II hypersensitivity reaction, 91, 92, 212
type III hypersensitivity reaction, 91, 92, 212
type IV hypersensitivity reaction, 91–3

ulcer, ulceration, 93, 137, 139, 169, 171, 172, 174, 175, 180, 182, 212
ultraviolet light, 15, 32, 166
unexpected drug reactions, 9
urates, uric acid, 36

urinary bladder, 36, 37, 38, 155, 157, 166, 172, 176
urinary tract, 66–8, 77
urine, 4, 6, 8, 88, 149, 172, 176, 180, 181
urine retention, 172
uroliths, 37
urticaria, 212
useful information for pathologists (when sending tumour biopsies to the lab), 182
uterus, 16, 17, 84, 155, 156

vaccine, vaccination, 7, 14, 67, 75, 77, 88, 178, 181
valves, of heart, 116,
valvular thrombosis, 142
variable regions, of antibodies/immunoglobins, 72–4
vascular permeability, see also permeability of capillaries, 46, 48
vascular phase of acute inflammation, 44, 56, 77
vasculitis, 54, 56, 92, 128, 138, 212
vasoconstriction, 128, 134, 135, 212
vasodilation, 46, 80, 90, 146–8, 213
vector, 213
vein(s), 116, 119, 139
vena cava, 116, 120
venom, 127, 138, 146, 148
venous bleeds, 116
venous circulation/outflow or drainage, 49, 116, 118, 148
ventricles, of heart, 116
venule, 116, 117, 119, 167
vertebral discs, 145
vesicle, 213
veterinary investigation officers, VIOs, 8
viraemia, 213
viral inclusions, 29, 38, 140, 141, 213
Virchow's triad, 213
virologist (s), 6
virulence, 213
virus(es), 6, 12, 14, 15, 29, 44, 66–9, 78, 79, 81, 84, 87, 88, 93, 166, 178
vitamin D toxicity, 35, 37
vitamin K, 132, 138, 139
vitamin K deficiency, 138
volvulus, 213
vomit, blood in, 172, 176, 180
vomiting, 176
von Willebrand factor, VWF, 139
von Willebrand's disease, 139
vulnerability (to disease), 16, 19, 66, 84, 87, 88, 93

Warfarin, 138
water, 50
weakness, 93
weight loss, wasting, 53, 55, 61, 176, 180
wet gangrene, 32, 35
wheal, 213
whelping, 20
white blood cells, 6, 13, 50, 63, 79, 176, 180
'white line' of acute inflammation, 45, 46
withers, 31
womb, see also uterus, 88
worms (parasitic), 7, 78
wound, 4, 103–7, 109, 177

yeasts, 6, 14